AF683247

THE PULMONARY ARTERY CATHETER

THE PULMONARY ARTERY CATHETER

Methodology & Clinical Applications

Edited by **Charles L. Sprung, M.D.**
Chief, Medical Intensive Care Unit
Veterans Administration Medical Center
Associate Professor of Medicine
University of Miami
School of Medicine
Miami, Florida

Contributors: **Joseph M. Civetta, M.D.**
Lawrence J. Jacobs, M.D.
Eric C. Rackow, M.D.
Bradley H. Ruben, D.O.
H. J. C. Swan, M.D., Ph.D., F.R.C.P.

UNIVERSITY PARK PRESS Baltimore

UNIVERSITY PARK PRESS
International Publishers in Medicine and Human Services
300 North Charles Street
Baltimore, Maryland 21201

Copyright © 1983 by University Park Press
Second Printing, August 1984

Typeset by Oberlin Printing Company

Manufactured in the United States of America by The Maple Press Company

This book is protected by copyright. All rights, including that of translation into other languages, are reserved. No part of this book may be reproduced, stored in a retrieval system, or transmitted, in any form or by any means, electronic, mechanical, photocopying, recording, or otherwise, without the prior written permission of the publisher.

Library of Congress Cataloging in Publication Data
Main entry under title:

The Pulmonary artery catheter.

Includes index.
1. Pulmonary artery—Catheterization. I. Sprung, Charles L. II. Civetta, Joseph M.
RC683.5.P84P8 1983 617'.412 82-24794
ISBN 0-8391-1808-2

Contents

Contributors

Joseph M. Civetta, M.D.
Professor and Chief
Division of Emergency Surgical Services
University of Miami School of Medicine/
Jackson Memorial Medical Center
Miami, Florida

Lawrence J. Jacobs, M.D.
Assistant Clinical Professor of Medicine
Division of Cardiology
University of Miami School of Medicine
Miami, Florida

Eric C. Rackow, M.D.
Professor and Vice Chairman
Department of Medicine
Chief, Division of Critical Care Medicine
Director, Center for Critical Care Medicine
University of Health Sciences/The Chicago Medical School
Chicago, Illinois

Bradley H. Ruben, D.O.
Assistant Professor of Anesthesiology, Neurological Surgery and Surgery
Director, Neurosurgical Intensive Care Unit
Co-Director, Surgical Intensive Care Unit
University of Miami School of Medicine/
Jackson Memorial Medical Center
Miami, Florida

Charles L. Sprung, M.D.
Chief, Medical Intensive Care Unit
Veterans Administration Medical Center
Associate Professor of Medicine
University of Miami School of Medicine
Miami, Florida

H. J. C. Swan, M.D., Ph.D., F.R.C.P.
Professor of Medicine
University of California (Los Angeles)
School of Medicine
Director of Cardiology
Cedars-Sinai Medical Center
Los Angeles, California

Preface

As is the case with any new drug or instrument, the pulmonary artery catheter was initially introduced with great promise and expectation. Not unexpectedly, over the next several years, complications (some fatal) were reported to occur secondary to pulmonary artery catheterization. Despite this fact, improvements in the capabilities of the pulmonary artery catheter have maintained its high rate of usage. Indeed, after more than a decade of use, Dr. Swan and colleagues' flotation catheter has truly revolutionized the care of the critically ill. Physiologic changes in a patient can now be observed at the bedside and treated appropriately. Unfortunately, pulmonary artery catheterization has never been shown to increase survival. Whether such a study could or should be done at this time is debatable. Surely an effort must be made to objectively define those patients who do clearly benefit from catheterization.

The present work represents an attempt to unify in one book the concepts and information available in the medical literature pertaining to pulmonary artery catheterization. It is meant for the student of hemodynamic monitoring. As we are all students in this area, this should include the in-training or practicing nurse, technician, therapist, or physician. Because of the different levels of knowledge of the aforementioned individuals and the many subspecialities involved in the care of patients requiring catheterization, my collaborators (two cardiologists, a surgeon, and an anesthesiologist,—all intensivists) and I have attempted to reach each group. The introduction is a perspective of the pulmonary artery catheter by Dr. Swan looking back and looking forward to the future. Chapter 1 contains the indications for catheterization. This information represents the criteria reported in the literature. Chapter 2 describes the methods and techniques for catheterization and pressure monitoring. Dr. Civetta has been using the catheter for many years, has previously reported some of his data and experience, and now gives his personal approach to insertion of the pulmonary artery catheter. Chapter 3 is a review of the current known complications of pulmonary artery catheterization. Guidelines to prevent these complications and to treat them once they occur are included. Chapter 4 is a discussion of the actual measurements made and calculations derived with the aid of the pulmonary artery catheter. Included is a discussion of the meaning of these variables. Finally, Chapter 5 contains selected patients with the typical disorders that require pulmonary artery catheterization. The authors have been extensively involved with patients with these disease states in a clinical and/or research setting. Each case is presented and the particular disorder and the benefits of hemodynamic monitoring in that particular patient are discussed. The term pulmonary artery catheter is used throughout the book as a uniform and "generic" description of the catheter.

The impetus to write this book came from my growing frustration and distress as I viewed the complacency of some physicians performing pulmonary artery catheterization. Some physicians would catheterize a patient when physical examination would suffice, whereas others would leave a patient's bedside immediately after the catheterization without utilizing the potential information the catheter could provide. It is hoped that this book will curtail these events and serve as a useful reference for those involved in the use of the pulmonary artery catheter.

Charles L. Sprung

Acknowledgments

The editor wishes to thank Joan Rodden, Rebecca Sprung, Peggy Pierce, Eileen Marcial, Yvonne Bisordi, Lorraine Scotto, Seymour Levine, and the Medical Library Staff of the Veterans Administration Medical Center for their technical assistance, and Dr. Michael Goldstein for his critical review of the book.

Finally, the editor would like to acknowledge our patients, students, hospital staff, house staff, and teachers who have been a source of inspiration and have made the pursuit of medicine more meaningful.

To my parents, brothers and sisters;
and especially to my wife Rebecca
and my children Elie, Nina, and Ari
who put up with me and my chosen profession.

Introduction

H. J. C. Swan

Dr. Sprung has performed a valuable service in bringing together current levels of knowledge on the processes and application of hemodynamic monitoring in the management of critically ill patients. He has also graciously provided me with the opportunity to overview the development of such procedures, which have expanded so rapidly in their application over the past 5 years.

The critically ill patient usually experiences severe cardiopulmonary distress, either because of primary disease of the heart or lungs, or because of disease of other organ systems. Whatever the fundamental cause of the problem, cardiopulmonary manifestations will frequently dominate the outcome in situations other than severe brain damage. The cardiovascular system, in particular, is vulnerable to rapid alterations in performance, and such alterations have a profound and potentially disastrous consequence on the preservation of overall bodily functions. However, such rapid changes in cardiovascular function are not necessarily accompanied by obvious clinical findings, and in particular, rapid deterioration (or improvement) in fundamental circulatory functions cannot be tracked with precision by attention to historical information and data obtained from conventional physical examination alone. True, the clinical differentiation from an individual experiencing normal good health from one who is moribund offers no particular diagnostic challenge. However, patients in the initial phase of cardiopulmonary illness may not appear to be seriously ill for several hours, whereas patients with disorders of other organ systems, trauma, sepsis, or coagulation disorders may succumb acutely from the effects of such processes on cardiopulmonary function.

Thus, the need for a careful and continued assessment of the functional state of the cardiovascular and pulmonary systems in critically ill patients has always been with us, but it has been only recently that formal clinical hemodynamic monitoring on a wide scale has become possible.

Historically, the development of diagnostic cardiac catheterization in the late 1940s and early 1950s allowed the application of the fundamental elements of cardiovascular physiology to clinical diagnosis and therapy. In particular, the significance of the levels of pressure in the heart and great vessels, the behavior of the peripheral vascular resistance and venous volume regulation was appreciated, and above all, the significance of the level of cardiac output, delivery of oxygen and removal of metabolic waste products became relevant in clinical terms. Of the greatest importance is the recognition that low cardiac output (less than 1.8 liters/min/m^2) may not be compatible with long survival (with the exception of chronic mitral stenosis). In fact, cardiac indices of 1.0 liters/min/m^2 are not compatible with survival beyond a few hours in the great majority of instances. Thus, relatively modest changes of cardiac output in this low range are highly relevant in terms of survival of the functioning organism.

Although these measurements could be made routinely in a diagnostic cardiac catheterization laboratory furnished with the appropriate radiologic equipment, their application at the bedside was prevented by several practical factors. The first of these was that critically ill patients could not be effectively moved to radiologic facilities for diagnostic cardiac catheterization procedures. Secondly, the monitoring procedures had to be applied at the bedside and in the common areas of ordinary bedside clinical care. Further, and perhaps most importantly, those personnel who provided true bedside care of the patient, the nurse, had to be extensively involved in the process and procedures of hemodynamic monitoring.

It must not be assumed that hemodynamic monitoring had not been practiced in the past. Indeed, in the experience of this writer while working at the Mayo Clinic, measurements of intra-arterial pressure, central venous pressure, heart rate and rhythm, and cardiac output, using Indocyanine green dye were carried out in the operating rooms of Dr. John Kirklin at the Mayo Clinic in 1954 and subsequently. However, the principal purpose of such studies was to determine optimal conditions for the application of the new techniques of extracorporeal circulatory support for open-heart surgery. A number of investigations by Moffitt, Theye and colleagues in anesthesiology pertained to the evaluation of appropriate anesthesia techniques in the same program.

From 1951, this author had the privilege of working under the rigorous guidance of Earl H. Wood, M.D., Ph.D., who instilled into his personnel—physician and technician alike—a healthy respect for the principles of biomedical instrumentation, the techniques of cardiac catheterization, and the rigorous analysis and application of the data derived therefrom. He also espoused the reasonable postulate that all such data should be relevant and should be obtained with minimal trauma and risk to the patient.

When faced with the challenge of understanding the processes of ischemic heart disease, this author had several of the above limitations in mind in the development of the flow-guided balloon-tipped cardiac catheter which, in association with Dr. William Ganz, bears his name. The principles of flexible catheters had been recognized by Dotter and by Bradley (1, 2). The availability of an existing latex balloon (Fogerty) resulted in a substitution for the original notion of a sail or parachute as the guidance device. The use of an obstructing balloon (Dotter) had been recognized to facilitate entry of a catheter into the pulmonary artery in the experimental animal (Lategola and Rahn) (3, 4).

Nevertheless, the author and his colleagues never anticipated the broad and general application of the balloon-flotation catheter for pressure measurement, the thermodilution measurement of cardiac output and the quantitation of systemic and pulmonary vascular resistance as other than a research tool.

Hemodynamic monitoring, therefore, is simply the application of the principles of cardiac catheterization in a bedside and clinical, as opposed to a specialized laboratory, setting. The initial double lumen catheter first described in the *New England Journal of Medicine* in 1970 (5) has undergone many modifications and can be obtained in various forms from several manufacturers. The data so obtained can be manipulated and presented in a manner useful to the health care personnel responsible for management of the critically ill. Although no carefully defined studies have established on a scientific basis the particular benefit of hemodynamic monitoring to the individual patient, it is reasonable to assume that a more precise and continuous knowledge of fundamental cardiovascular parameters would allow for more optimal decisions as to therapy, if not today, then certainly in the future. It is the impression of a wide variety of physicians, however, that substantially sicker patients are now being subjected to needed surgery than in the past, and that fewer patients are being denied surgery because of cardiovascular, pulmonary, or other short-term contraindications. Of course, hemodynamic monitoring has little to offer a patient in the absence of an effective therapeutic plan. If the root cause of an illness or disorder cannot be eradicated or modified, or if no intervention is considered effective, then hemodynamic monitoring has no place in the management of such patients.

To project into the future, it appears likely that hemodynamic monitoring techniques, including the use of the flotation catheter and the direct measurement of intra-arterial pressure, will remain a fundamental component of the management of the critically ill for many years to come. Competing techniques appear to have fair to poor absolute correlations, little predictive value in the individual patient and reflect small or moderate, yet clinically highly significant changes in circulatory parameters poorly.

The developing subspecialty of Critical Care Medicine is an appropriate discipline in which to place responsibility for hemodynamic monitoring. The simple placement of a balloon flotation catheter and an arterial line as a technical procedure alone does not constitute effective hemodynamic monitoring, and the abandonment of the patient by a physician, once lines have been placed, appears to be an act of professional neglect, unless appropriate application of the derived data to the care of the patient is included as part of that responsibility. However, rigorous programs of training in hemodynamic monitoring must be developed with appropriate standards. The current system of "learning by doing" is neither firmly nor rationally based. In many instances, "experienced" physicians have learned more through the ignorance and sometimes slipshod methods of their house staff predecessors than from individuals disciplined in laboratory procedures and physiological determinations. In fact, the rather cavalier attitude of many physicians in regard to hemodynamic monitoring is undoubtedly partly responsible for the continued incidence of important, but avoidable, complications of these techniques. In the future, I see that these will become more specialized and in the domain of one group within a given hospital complex; namely, the intensivist of the future.

REFERENCES

1. Dotter, C. T., and Straube, K. R. 1962. Flow guided cardiac catheterization. Am. J. Roentgenol. Rad. Ther. Nuclear Med. 88:27-30.
2. Bradley, R. D. 1964. Diagnostic right heart catheterization with miniature catheters in severely ill patients. Lancet 2:941-942.
3. Dotter, C. T., and Lukas, D. S. 1951. Acute cor pulmonale: An experimental study utilizing a special cardiac catheter. Am. J. Physiol. 164:254-262.
4. Lategola, M., and Rahn, H. 1953. A self-guiding catheter for cardiac and pulmonary arterial catheterization and occlusion. Proc. Soc. Exp. Biol. Med. 84:667-668.
5. Swan, H. J. C., Ganz, W., Forrester, J., Marcus, H., Diamond, G., and Chonette, D. 1970. Catheterization of the heart in man with use of a flow-directed balloon-tipped catheter. N. Engl. J. Med. 283:447-451.

Section I

Methodology

Chapter 1

Indications for Pulmonary Artery Catheterization

Charles L. Sprung and Lawrence J. Jacobs

For she hath cast down many wounded,
yea, all her slain are a mighty host.
Proverbs 7:26

"For she hath cast down many wounded" refers to a disciple who has not attained the qualifications to decide questions of law and yet decides them; whereas "yea, all her slain are a mighty host" refers to a disciple who has attained the qualifications to decide questions of law but does not decide them (1). An analogy may be drawn to hemodynamic monitoring. Inappropriate use of a balloon-tipped flow-directed catheter and, conversely, the omission of catheterization when an indication exists may lead to morbidity and mortality. The widespread popularity of hemodynamic monitoring has led to the indiscriminate use of the pulmonary artery catheter in many clinical circumstances (2). In other situations, the flotation catheter remains under-utilized, even for conservative indications (3). Some respected experts have practiced unaided clinical observation, whereas others have emphasized the importance of aggressive invasive monitoring. Unfortunately, prospective studies to determine the specific indications for pulmonary artery catheterization have not been performed. Therefore, physicians must weigh the potential benefits against the risks in each individual patient before performing a bedside pulmonary catheterization. This is especially true of critically ill patients with pre-existing cardiovascular or pulmonary disease or increased susceptibility to bleeding and infection. These patients typically have the greatest need for catheterization, and yet are the most prone to the complications. One must always remember that complications do occur and that they may be fatal.

Clinical findings often lag behind or fail to reflect hemodynamic data (4). Therefore, the treatment of patients by clinical criteria alone may cause radical, unwanted changes in the heart rate, preload, afterload, and contractility. Although these alterations of the determinants of myocardial oxygen consumption may not be clinically apparent, they may have profound detrimental effects on the critically ill patient, especially a patient with acute myocardial infarction. Consequently, the dynamic information provided by invasive pulmonary artery catheterization may indeed constitute a "conservative" approach to therapy in these patients.

The performance of bedside right heart catheterization will depend on factors other than the appropriate medical indication. A commitment must be made to purchase expensive and durable equipment and to provide specially trained physicians, nurses, and technicians on a continuous basis. Physicians performing catheterizations must recognize the indications and contraindications, the techniques employed, the complications and their recognition, and the methods to avoid and to treat the complications of catheterization. Physicians and nurses should be familiar with the entire system including the monitors, transducers, and catheter. They should be capable of trouble shooting technical problems and of recognizing and differentiating the various pressure tracings. The aforementioned prerequisites will assure the acquisition of accurate and reproducible information with minimal risk. Unfortunately, pulmonary artery catheters continue to be inserted without the satisfaction of these prerequisites. Under these circumstances data are often inaccurate, information is interpreted incorrectly, and inappropriate therapeutic interventions are instituted. Patients themselves may be ignored so that the staff can observe their "numbers." The pulmonary artery catheter can provide critical insight into the pathophysiology of various disease states. This information should complement but never replace common sense and good clinical judgment.

Pulmonary artery catheterization is performed to establish a diagnosis or to determine the initial or ongoing therapies to be administered. Catheterization should not be performed if similar information can be obtained by noninvasive means. Invasive monitoring should be used only if a question is asked and the answer obtained by catheterization can change the diagnostic or therapeutic decisions to be made. There are reports of physicians who have refused to believe the information provided by the pulmonary artery catheter and have treated their patients clinically to the detriment of their patients (5). If the same actions will be taken despite the results of catheterization, there is no need to subject a patient to this potentially dangerous procedure.

The balloon-tipped catheter enables one to measure central venous pressure, pulmonary artery pressures, cardiac output, and mixed venous blood samples. Thus, the physiologic data to evaluate pulmonary and right and left ventricular function are available in various disease states. The major indications for pulmonary artery catheterization are listed in Table 1.1. As noted previously, the potential benefits of catheterization must outweigh the risks. Various physicians may define indications liberally, whereas others will be more stringent. Table 1.1 represents the indications most frequently noted in the medical literature. A more complete discussion of the measurements and calculations obtained with the pulmonary artery catheter and their importance in various disease states is found in the Clinical Applications section (Chapters 4 and 5).

I. COMPLICATED MYOCARDIAL INFARCTION OR MYOCARDIAL ISCHEMIA

Most patients with acute myocardial infarction (AMI) do not require bedside catheterization and do well, despite the presence of tachycardia, hypertension, or pulmonary congestion. Patients suffering complicated myocardial infarctions have a higher mortality rate than those patients with uncompli-

Table 1.1. Indications for pulmonary artery catheterization

I. Complicated myocardial infarction or myocardial ischemia
    A. Hypotension
    B. Congestive heart failure
    C. Sinus tachycardia
    D. Hypertension
    E. Acute mitral regurgitation
    F. Ventricular septal defect
    G. Pericardial tamponade
    H. Right ventricular infarction
    I. Evaluate pharmacologic agents
    J. Assess interventions to decrease myocardial infarct size
II. Shock
III. Pulmonary
    A. Cardiogenic pulmonary edema
    B. Respiratory failure
    C. Respiratory distress of unknown cause
IV. Assess intravascular volume
V. Vasodilation
VI. Surgical
    A. High-risk patient
    B. Proposed surgical procedure
        1. Surgery associated with a high mortality
        2. Anticipated large volume requirements
    C. Postoperative complication
VII. Pediatric
VIII. Routine cardiac catheterization
IX. Miscellaneous

cated courses, and often require some therapeutic intervention. Most patients with complicated AMI have, in fact, received some treatment prior to catheterization. Certain complications necessitate immediate catheterization. Patients with AMI may have disparate right and left ventricular function, and the pulmonary artery wedge pressure (PWP) more accurately reflects left ventricular function than does the central venous pressure (CVP) (6). In these patients, right heart catheterization provides an accurate assessment of prognosis and left ventricular function as reflected by both filling pressure and cardiac output. Therapy aimed at decreasing myocardial oxygen demand and increasing oxygen delivery guided by continuous hemodynamic monitoring, will hopefully salvage border zones of ischemia.

A. Hypotension

The majority of patients with AMI and hypotension (systolic blood pressure less than 90 mm Hg) are hypovolemic and require volume infusion; these patients are not truly in cardiogenic shock. Fluid must be administered cautiously to a patient with a noncompliant ventricle to avoid pulmonary edema. Therefore, if initial, empirical attempts at fluid resuscitation fail to increase cardiac output and blood pressure, catheterization is performed. Optimal filling pressure in these patients ranges from 14 to 18 mm Hg as measured by PWP (7). A Starling curve can be constructed for each patient to precisely determine an optimal PWP. Patients remaining hypotensive after volume expansion are often in cardiogenic shock and exhibit clinical signs of hypoperfusion. Their cardiac indices are typically less than 2.2 liters/min/m^2 and they require inotropes and/or vasodilators.

B. Congestive Heart Failure

Patients with clinical evidence of congestive heart failure (gallops, rales, etc.) but without shock, usually do not require catheterization. If standard therapy (usually oxygen, morphine sulfate, and furosemide) fails, however, catheterization is performed. Profound diuresis without the measurement of ventricular filling pressures can lead to hypovolemia and even shock. After catheterization, further diuresis or vasodilator therapy (especially in the presence of hypertension) may be indicated.

C. Sinus Tachycardia

Because heart rate is a major determinant of myocardial oxygen consumption, tachycardia in patients with AMI must be aggressively evaluated. Treatable causes such as chest pain, anxiety, congestive heart failure, infection, and pericarditis should be considered. Typically, sedation and/or analgesia are all that is required. If sinus tachycardia in the range of 120-150 beats/min persists despite adequate treatment of these etiologies, either hypovolemia or extensive myocardial damage is probably present. Determining the exact cause and the appropriate treatment may be difficult even for the most experienced clinician. Right heart catheterization will enable the physician to appropriately volume resuscitate the hypovolemic patient or diurese or vasodilate the hypervolemic patient. Therapy should lower the heart rate and thereby decrease myocardial oxygen consumption.

D. Hypertension

Arterial blood pressure is also a determinant of myocardial oxygen consumption. Therefore, hypertension (BP $>$ 145/95 mm Hg) complicating myocardial infarction or ischemia may be detrimental. Hypertension is not an uncommon problem in patients with AMI. Analgesia (morphine sulfate) and sedation (diazepam) can usually normalize blood pressure in most patients. If hypertension persists, diuretics, nitrates, and/or nitroprusside are used. These therapeutic modalities are frequently used empirically, without pulmonary artery catheterization. Many physicians believe, however, that therapy can be more precisely titrated in the patient with hypertension by means of a flotation catheter.

E. Acute Mitral Regurgitation

F. Ventricular Septal Defect

The discovery of a new systolic murmur after an acute myocardial infarction should suggest either acute mitral regurgitation or rupture of the interventricular septum. Unfortunately, the features of the murmur are often nonspecific, and the diagnosis can not be made on clinical grounds. Pulmonary artery catheterization is performed in these patients. Blood samples are obtained sequentially from the superior vena cava, right atrium, right ventricle, and pulmonary artery as the balloon catheter is advanced. The presence of a significant "step-up" in right ventricular or pulmonary artery oxygen saturation (a difference of greater than one volume percent between the right atrium and right ventricle or pulmonary artery) is diagnostic of ventricular septal rupture. Large "V" waves in the pulmonary artery wedge pressure or retrograde V waves in the pulmonary artery pressure wave, on the other hand, reflect acute mitral regurgitation (8).

The treatment of acute mitral regurgitation and ventricular septal rupture is somewhat similar and the pulmonary artery catheter helps guide therapy which may include diuretics, vasodilators, inotropic support, intra-aortic balloon counterpulsation or surgery.

G. Pericardial Tamponade

Cardiac tamponade is characterized by a rising venous pressure, a falling arterial blood pressure, and a small quiet heart (9). Unfortunately, these criteria apply to tamponade of rapid onset and may not always hold true.

Paradoxical pulse is present in the majority of patients. Cardiac tamponade is commonly related to trauma, infection or neoplastic disease. However, tamponade may occur in patients with AMI, especially in those who are anticoagulated. The diagnosis is often apparent by clinical, radiographic, and echo-cardiographic criteria and pericardiocentesis may be accomplished without catheterization. Catheterization may be particularly important in determining the hemodynamic significance of a pericardial effusion, especially in patients with myocardial infarction or ischemia. Catheterization is the only way to definitively establish the diagnosis, assess its severity, and monitor the effects of pericardiocentesis. Characteristically, the diastolic pressures of the right atrium, right ventricle, pulmonary artery, and left ventricle (reflected by the pulmonary artery wedge pressure) are of equal magnitude and similar contour (4). The pulse pressure is narrow and the wave form characteristically demonstrates a diastolic plateau with a paradoxical inspiratory rise. Concordant right atrial and PWP, however, do not always signify cardiac tamponade. Patients with right ventricular infarction may also have near equalization of right-and left-sided pressures.

H. Right Ventricular Infarction

Right ventricular infarction is often suspected when hemodynamics suggest disproportionately severe right ventricular dysfunction. Right atrial pressure equal to or greater than left ventricular filling pressure has been noted to be the characteristic hemodynamic finding of right ventricular infarction (10). In addition, elevated systemic venous pressure, absence of pulmonary edema, low cardiac output, and frequently arterial hypotension are present (10). Right ventricular infarction invariably coexists with left ventricular infarction. In fact, right ventricular damage may be present in 19-43% of patients with acute inferior myocardial infarction. Hemodynamic monitoring may have been performed for another complication of myocardial infarction and right ventricular infarction discovered by chance. Occasionally, adequate perfusion will be impossible without high right-sided filling pressures in patients with right ventricular infarction. The diagnosis of right ventricular infarction is based on disproportionately severe right ventricular dysfunction, which is not, however, specific for this disorder. Other etiologies of right ventricular failure, such as pulmonary embolism, chronic obstructive pulmonary disease (higher pulmonary vascular resistances are usually present), and others must be ruled out. In addition, elevated systemic venous pressure, hypotension, paradoxical pulse, and even equilibration of diastolic pressures may be present in right ventricular infarction; these findings may be misinterpreted as representing cardiac tamponade or constrictive pericardial disease. A well-preserved and steep right atrial Y descent and a right ventricular pressure tracing showing an early diastolic dip and plateau configuration, which are also found in patients with constrictive pericarditis, may be observed in patients with right ventricular infarction (10). Noninvasive examinations (echocardiography, scanning) can usually differentiate the dilated and poorly contracting right-sided chambers of right ventricular infarction from the small, vigorously contracting chambers of cardiac tamponade and constrictive pericarditis.

I. Evaluate Pharmacologic Agents

As noted previously, many patients with complicated myocardial infarction require diuretics, vasodilators, inotropes, and/or vasopressors. In order to accurately monitor response to therapy, pulmonary artery catheterization is often required.

J. Assess Interventions to Decrease Myocardial Infarct Size

In addition to pharmacologic agents used to optimize physiologic parameters and decrease infarct size, other interventions, such as intra-aortic balloon counterpulsation and experimental modalities, may require evaluation by hemodynamic monitoring.

II. SHOCK

Shock is defined as a systolic blood pressure less than 90 mm Hg on successive determinations (or 50 mm Hg less than the baseline systolic blood pressure in previously hypertensive patients) with signs of inadequate tissue perfusion. Hypoperfusion is characterized by an abnormal mental status (lethargy, stupor, or coma), oliguria (urine output less than 20 ml/hr), and lactate production. The various types of shock include hypovolemic, cardiogenic, distributive (septic), and obstructive etiologies. Volume infusion is often the initial treatment of the various types of shock. A peripheral or CVP catheter is usually inserted to initiate fluid therapy. If volume infusion does not quickly reverse the shock state, pulmonary artery catheterization is indicated. This is especially imperative in patients with disparate right and left ventricular function or elevated central venous pressures. The flow-directed catheter can provide both diagnostic and therapeutic usefulness. Careful volume resuscitation is guided by the measurement of left ventricular filling pressure (PWP), cardiac output, and clinical examination. The effect of inotropic and vasopressor agents can also be observed.

III. PULMONARY

Cardiac and respiratory failure often coexist in the same patient. The pulmonary artery catheter helps differentiate the cardiac (elevated PWP, decreased cardiac output) and pulmonary (increased pulmonary artery diastolic pressure—PWP gradient, increased pulmonary veno-arterial admixture) disorders that may be difficult if not impossible to distinguish clinically.

A. Cardiogenic Pulmonary Edema

In addition to patients with AMI, patients with valvular disorders, hypertensive heart disease, cardiomyopathies, myocardial ischemia, and tachyarrhythmias may also present with pulmonary edema. As noted in patients with AMI, most patients are treated with agents that decrease preload; these patients do not require catheterization. The rare patient with pulmonary edema that persists despite intensive therapy requires catheterization. The flow-directed catheter provides an evaluation of left ventricular filling pressures and a continuous guide to further treatment.

B. Respiratory Failure

A frequent cause of mortality in the intensive care unit is noncardiogenic pulmonary edema or the adult respiratory distress syndrome (ARDS). The diagnosis is based on physical and radiologic evidence of bilateral pulmonary infiltrates consistent with edema, hypoxemia ($pO_2/FIO_2 < 160$), normal left ventricular filling pressure (PWP), and if obtainable, increased edema fluid to serum protein or colloid osmotic pressure ratios (ratio > 0.7) (11). Most patients have a history of a predisposing factor (shock, trauma, sepsis, etc.) and have hearts of normal size. The pulmonary artery catheter is required in these patients to exclude the diagnosis of cardiac edema and to guide the use of positive end-expiratory pressure (PEEP). Many authorities perform right heart catheterization in patients with any type of respiratory failure who require 5-10 cm/H_2O of PEEP;others catheterize patients even before this criterion is satisfied. With the aid of the pulmonary artery catheter, the influence of PEEP on cardiac output, oxygen transport, and intrapulmonary shunting can be monitored (12). In this way, optimal PEEP can be established for a given patient.

Catheterization is also occasionally used for patients with central nervous system depression of ventilation (overdose or others). Problems such as persistent hypotension are the usual reasons for catheterization.

C. Respiratory Distress of Unknown Cause

As noted, situations occur in which the relative contributions of cardiac or pulmonary disease to respiratory distress is unclear by clinical examination. Typically, the patient exhibits rales and/or rhonchi on auscultation. The pulmonary artery catheter can help differentiate congestive heart failure from pneumonia, pulmonary emboli, ARDS, or chronic pulmonary disorders.

IV. ASSESS INTRAVASCULAR VOLUME

Many patients have heart, lung, and renal diseases that do not allow accurate determinations of volume status based on clinical criteria alone. These patients may have clinical or roentgenographic evidence of congestive heart failure or elevated central venous pressure, but require fluid therapy for hypotension, hyperalimentation, severe burns, trauma, or transfusion requirements. The pulmonary artery catheter permits an exact determination of left ventricular filling pressure which allows appropriate therapy with fluid, diuretics, inotropes, vasodilators, or vasopressors.

V. VASODILATION

Cardiac failure secondary to AMI or ischemia, valvular disease, or cardiomyopathy may be manifest by reduced cardiac output and/or elevated pulmonary and systemic venous pressures. Vasodilator therapy has become a standard form of treatment in the last decade. Short-acting intravenous preparations (sodium nitroprusside, nitroglycerin, and trimethaphan) are used in patients with AMI and pump failure. Hemodynamic monitoring is obviously required in these patients. Many patients with chronic cardiac failure receive oral vasodilator therapy (nitrates, hydralazine, prazosin) as outpatients without hemodynamic monitoring. To determine the predominant abnormality (preload versus afterload) and the optimal dosages of medication, however, pulmonary artery catheterization may be helpful even in the patient without AMI or acute ischemia. Changes in left ventricular filling pressure, cardiac output, systemic vascular resistance, and systemic blood pressure guide proper therapy.

VI. SURGICAL

Hemodynamic monitoring may be invaluable when compromised patients are challenged with the considerable stresses of anesthesia and surgery. Preoperative, intraoperative, and/or postoperative monitoring may therefore be necessary.

A. High-Risk Patient

Major operations may precipitate left ventricular failure, myocardial or mesenteric infarction, or acute tubular necrosis in patients with marginal cardiovascular reserve. Del Guercio and Cohn have noted that standard preoperative assessment of the elderly for surgery is often inadequate (13). Hemodynamic monitoring revealed mild or moderate physiologic abnormalities in 64% of patients, and advanced defects making patients unacceptable risks for major surgery in 23% of patients (13). Therefore, hemodynamic monitoring may be especially useful in the elderly and in the patient with underlying cardiovascular or respiratory disease. Criteria for defining which patients are at high risk and who may benefit from preoperative monitoring have not yet been established.

B. Proposed Surgical Procedure

Patients undergoing extensive surgery associated with increased operative risk and mortality may benefit from hemodynamic monitoring. This is especially true of patients with compromised cardiac or pulmonary function, but may also apply to those patients without underlying disease. In addition, patients undergoing surgery with anticipated large blood loss, massive transfusions, or large volume requirements may also benefit from pulmonary artery catheterization and monitoring. Patients requiring the following operations may therefore benefit from hemodynamic monitoring: intrathoracic operations; major surgery on the aorta or cerebral blood vessels; hepatic and intestinal surgery; surgery for multiple trauma; pelvic exenteration; or operations requiring induced hypotension anesthesia. Monitoring pulmonary artery pressure for detection and treatment of air embolism during seated neurosurgical procedures may also be helpful (14).

Routine right heart catheterization has been performed for patients undergoing cardiac surgery (valve replacement or coronary artery bypass) in some centers. Mangano has tried to delineate the indications for pulmonary artery catheterization in patients undergoing coronary artery surgery (15). He found that CVP and PWP correlated well in patients who had ejection fractions greater than 0.5 without angiographically demonstrable ventricular dyssynergy. CVP and PWP did not correlate in patients with ejection fractions less than 0.4 or with dyssynergy. This latter group, unlike the former, would therefore benefit from PWP determinations rather than CVP measurements (15). It is unfortunate that there are few studies delineating subgroups of patients likely to benefit from catheterization in other surgical procedures or disease states. Before performing pulmonary artery catheterization in any surgical patient, one must justify the need for that particular patient. Not all patients, even those with heart disease, require hemodynamic monitoring for all surgical procedures.

C. Postoperative Complications

Complications may occur after surgery that require pulmonary artery catheterization. These include myocardial infarction or ischemia, cardiogenic or septic shock, respiratory failure, cardiac tamponade, and others.

VII. PEDIATRIC

Smaller and more flexible catheters, including catheters for measuring cardiac output by thermodilution, are available for use in pediatric patients. The same indications apply to the pediatric population. In addition, the balloon-tipped flotation catheter has been helpful in the cardiac catheterization laboratory for infants and children with congenital abnormalities (16). These include 1) catheterization of children in whom the exact anatomy and position of the cardiac chambers are not known; 2) manipulation of the catheter into heart chambers and blood vessels not easily approached by conventional means, such as entry into the pulmonary artery from the left or common ventricle or entry into the aorta from the right or common ventricle in transposition of the great vessels; 3) catheter passage through an intra-atrial communication into the left atrium, left ventricle, and aorta to avoid retrograde arterial catheterization and an arteriotomy; and 4) obtaining pulmonary artery wedge pressure measurements in patients in whom these measurements would otherwise be difficult to obtain.

Caution must obviously be used when the catheter is positioned in the systemic arterial circuit, as the balloon can occlude a major vessel. Pressure monitoring and deflation of the balloon to maintain the catheter's correct position is therefore extremely important in the systemic as well as the pulmonary vascular system.

VIII. ROUTINE CARDIAC CATHETERIZATION

Right heart catheterization of the right ventricle and pulmonary artery can often be performed with a lower incidence of serious arrhythmias and in less time by using the balloon-tipped flow-directed catheter. It is, therefore, not surprising that the balloon-tipped catheter has been used routinely in many cardiac catheterization laboratories.

IX. MISCELLANEOUS

Other indications for pulmonary artery catheterization include patients with decompensated cirrhosis, peritonitis, or trauma who require central catheterization. These patients and probably many other critically ill patients have disparate right and left heart pressures (17).

In addition to the usual functions of the flow-directed balloon-tipped catheter, the multipurpose pulmonary artery catheter (Edwards Laboratories) also provides the capability for atrial (A), ventricular (V), or A-V sequential pacing, overdrive suppression of atrial or ventricular arrhythmias, and intracavitary electrocardiograms to diagnose complex arrhythmias (18). Unfortunately the usefulness of this multipurpose catheter has not been great because the atrial and ventricular electrodes function only when properly positioned. Therefore, this catheter can not be used in patients with enlarged hearts because the proper positioning of the electrodes is usually impossible. Also, the electrodes function only when the catheter tip has been advanced to the pulmonary artery and not before. Pulmonary angiography can also be performed through a balloon-tipped catheter and may help in the diagnosis of pulmonary emboli (19).

As important as it is to review indications for catheterization, it is equally important to consider contraindications. Bedside pulmonary artery catheterization has been extremely useful in the most critically ill patients. These patients who were once considered too ill for catheterization have tolerated the procedure well and appear to benefit most from the information gleaned. Unfortunately, the incidence of complications also increases in these seriously ill patients. Therefore, despite the fact that there are no absolute contraindications to the procedure, there are certainly relative contraindications. Patients with coagulopathies and an increased incidence of bleeding should be approached with great caution, especially if a percutaneous approach to catheterization is employed. If catheterization is considered essential, a peripheral cutdown of a brachial vein or, if necessary, a percutaneous internal jugular vein approach (which is at least accessible to compression) should be performed. Subclavian and femoral approaches should be avoided. Immunocompromised patients with granulocytopenia have increased risks of infection, and catheterization of any type should be avoided. In addition, all concurrent conditions whose correction might improve the safety of the catheterization should be corrected. These include electrolyte abnormalities, hypoxemia, acidosis, anemia, ventricular irritability, hypotension, hypertension, congestive heart failure, digitalis toxicity, febrile illnesses, coagulopathies, and others. These abnormalities should certainly be corrected prior to elective catheterization. Unfortunately, some of these abnormalities may themselves constitute the indication for catheterization and may not be correctable until after catheterization. The physician's decision regarding catheterization of these patients is even more difficult. One must weigh the increased risks of catheterization against the importance of the information to be obtained.

The use of the pulmonary artery catheter will certainly change as greater technical advances are made in catheter design and hemodynamic monitoring in general. Physicians with different backgrounds in training will probably always have more liberal or conservative approaches to the use of the catheter. The most appropriate indication for pulmonary artery catheterization has been stated by Dr. Swan (20) as "any situation in which a physician would consider placing a central venous pressure line for the purpose of cardiovascular monitoring."

REFERENCES

1. Talmud, Tractate Sotah, 22A.
2. Dalen, J. E. 1979. Bedside hemodynamic monitoring. (Editorial). N. Engl. J. Med. 301:1176-1178.
3. Deming, W. M. 1980. Hazards of pulmonary artery catheterization. N. Engl. J. Med. 302:808.
4. Forrester, J. S., Diamond, G., Chatterjee, K., and Swan, H. J. C. 1976. Medical therapy of acute myocardial infarction by application of hemodynamic subsets. N. Engl. J. Med. 295:1356-1362, 1404-1413.

5. Quinn, K., and Quebbeman, E. J. 1981. Pulmonary artery pressure monitoring in the surgical intensive care unit. Arch. Surg. 116:872-876.
6. Forrester, J. S., Diamond, G., McHugh, T. J., and Swan, H. J. C. 1971. Filling pressures in the right and left sides of the heart in acute myocardial infarction. N. Engl. J. Med. 285:190-193.
7. Crexells, C., Chatterjee, K., Forrester, J. S., Dikshit, K., and Swan, H. J. C. 1973. Optimal level of filling pressure in the left side of the heart in acute myocardial infarction. N. Engl. J. Med. 289:1264-1266.
8. Meister, S. G., and Helfant, R. H. 1972. Rapid bedside differentiation of ruptured interventricular septum from acute mitral insufficiency. N. Engl. J. Med. 287:1024-1025.
9. Guberman, B. A., Fowler, N. O., Engel, P. J., Gueron, M., and Allen, J. M. 1981. Cardiac tamponade in medical patients. Circulation 64:633-640.
10. Lorell, B., Leinbach, R. C., Pohost, G. M., Gold, H. K., Dinsmore, R. E., Hutter, A. M., Pastore, J. O., and Desanctis, R. W. 1979. Right ventricular infarction: Clinical diagnosis and differentiation from cardiac tamponade and pericardial constriction. Am. J. Cardiol. 43:465-471.
11. Sprung, C. L., Rackow, E. C., Fein, I. A., Jacob, A. I., and Isikoff, S. K. 1981. The spectrum of pulmonary edema: Differentiation of cardiogenic, intermediate and noncardiogenic forms of pulmonary edema. Am. Rev. Respir. Dis. 124:718-722.
12. Suter, P. M., Fairley, H. B., and Isenberg, M. D. 1975. Optimum end-expiratory airway pressure in patients with acute pulmonary failure. N. Engl. J. Med. 292:284-289.
13. Del Guercio, L. R. M., and Cohn, J. D. 1980. Monitoring operative risk in the elderly. JAMA 243:1350-1355.
14. Marshall, W. K., and Bedford, R. F. 1980. Use of a pulmonary-artery catheter for detection and treatment of venous air embolism. Anesthesiology 52:131-134.
15. Mangano, D. T. 1980. Monitoring pulmonary arterial pressure in coronary artery disease. Anesthesiology 53:364-370.
16. Ganz, W., and Swan, H. J. C. 1980. Balloon-tipped flow-directed catheters. In W. Grossman (ed.). Cardiac Catheterization and Angiography, pp. 78-86. Lea and Febiger, Philadelphia.
17. Civetta, J. M., and Gabel, J. C. 1972. Flow directed pulmonary artery catheterization in surgical patients: Indications and modifications of technic. Ann. Surg. 176:753-756.
18. Swan, H. J. C., and Ganz, W. 1975. Use of balloon flotation catheters in critically ill patients. Surg. Clin. North Am. 55:501-520.
19. Wilson, J. E., and Bynum, L. J. 1976. An improved pulmonary angiographic technique using a balloon-tipped catheter. Am. Rev. Respir. Dis. 114:1137-1144.
20. Swan, H. J. C., 1975. Balloon flotation catheters: Their use in hemodynamic monitoring in clinical practice. (Editorial). JAMA 233:865-867.

Chapter 2

Pulmonary Artery Catheter Insertion

Joseph M. Civetta

The quantum jump in information gathered using invasive pulmonary artery catheterization to monitor cardiovascular performance also requires that the user must acquire information beyond the physiologic implications of the data in order to insure that the information derived is accurate and can be used with confidence in interpreting the clinical situation. The relevant information encompasses an understanding of the electronic monitoring system, methods of calibrating, catheter design features, standardization of insertion techniques and equipment, the significance of the pressure and cardiac output measurements, and finally, an understanding of the pitfalls and errors that are possible and remedies that are available.

I. EQUIPMENT AND PREPARATION

A. Requirements for Electronic Monitoring

The generation of the pulsatile waveform viewed on an electronic monitor is a complex physical process. Pulsatile flow created by cardiac contraction to achieve forward movement is accomplished by episodic injection of the stroke volume into the elastic vascular system. During the period of ventricular ejection, pressure in the system rises and is accommodated by the elastic properties of both the pulmonary and systemic arteries. The pulmonary arterial system differs from the systemic arterial system in that its resistance is much lower so that, despite the fact that a similar stroke volume is ejected from both the right and left ventricles, pressure in the pulmonary arterial system is much lower. When cardiac ejection ceases, flow is continued, induced by the energy stored during the stretching of the arteries. Measurements of the pulmonary arterial system, therefore, must be precise because the pressures generated are much lower than systemic arterial pressure. This pulsatile flow is then transformed into a to and fro fluid movement in the intravascular catheter. When the catheter is connected to a transducer, the fluid motion in the vascular system is transformed into an electrical signal. The transducer is an electromechanical device (Figure 2.1) comprised of a fluid-filled dome which is applied to a sensitive diaphragm. Because fluid is not compressible, the to and fro motion of the fluid is directly transmitted to the diaphragm and results in periodic motion. On the undersurface of the diaphragm, a strain gauge, which is a system of variable resistances, is connected to an electrical component called a *Wheatstone bridge*. The Wheatstone bridge is a rectangular structure (Figure 2.2) com-

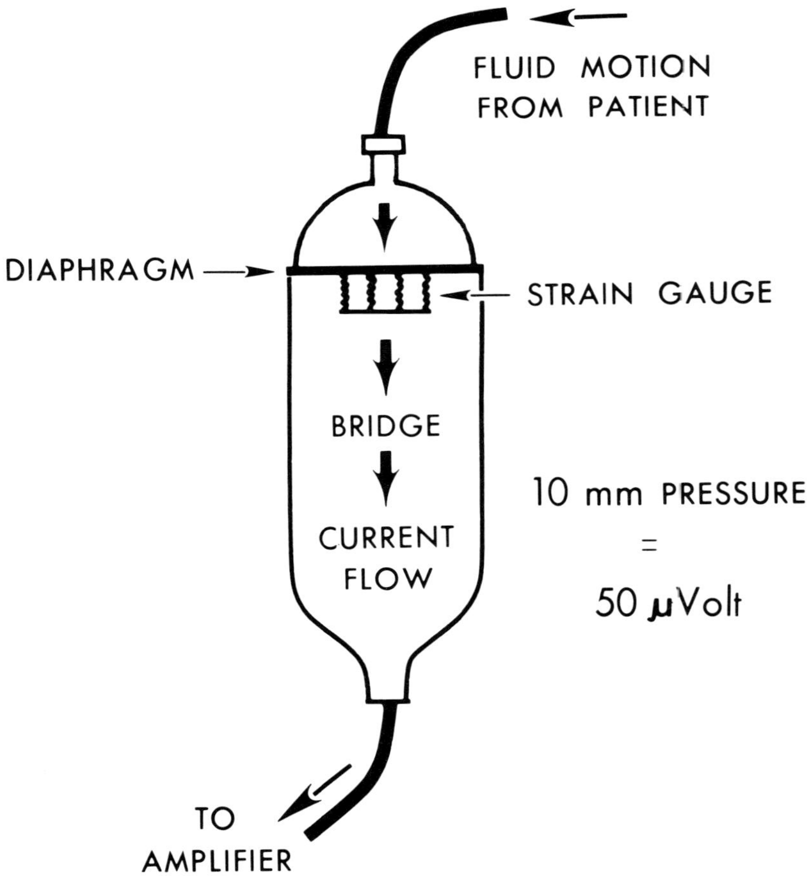

Figure 2.1. Diagramatic representation of a blood pressure transducer. The transducer changes energy of one form into another. In this instance, the energy generated by the pulsatile flow against the transducer diaphragm is transformed into an electrical current.

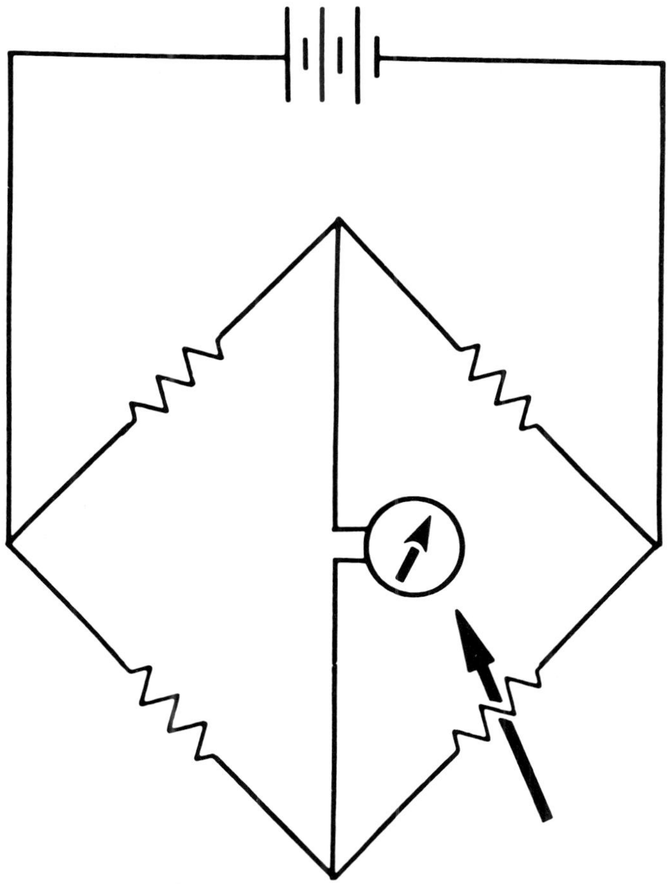

Figure 2.2. The Wheatstone Bridge. Note that there are three electrical resistances incorporated into the circuit which are calibrated in terms of ohms. The fourth resistance, denoted by the arrow crossing the serrated line, is variable and, when properly adjusted, there will be no electrical output from the bridge.

posed of three fixed electrical resistances and the variable resistance of the diaphragm. When a Wheatstone bridge is balanced, the variable resistance is adjusted so that the product of two arms is equalled by the product of the remaining two resistances. When the variable resistance changes such as when motion is imparted to the diaphragm by fluid flow, the Wheatstone bridge becomes "unbalanced." This induces an electrical current in the system which is delivered to an amplifying circuit in the monitor. Most transducers will produce an electrical signal of approximately 50 microvolts for every 10 mm of pressure applied to the diaphragm of its transducer. The monitor then amplifies the signal by approximately 5-10 times in order to produce a visible tracing on the screen. We must next consider the electronic characteristics of the monitor in order to reproduce this signal faithfully. There are four major considerations which involve the intravascular catheter, connecting tubing, transducer, and electronic monitor: 1) frequency response, 2) relative natural frequency; 3) damping; 4) catheter whip artifact (1). We encounter limitations in frequency response in two analogous situations. The familiar dog whistle, which is inaudible to our ears but readily heard by the dog, indicates that the frequency response of the canine ear is more sensitive than ours. Another example is found in listening to a high quality symphonic recording on a child's phonograph. It sounds tinny and lacks the lush fullness of sound heard in the concert hall. On an expensive stereo system with a frequency response capable of reproducing the highest and lowest sounds, however, a remarkable increase in the quality of the sound is evident. Biologic signals, just as sound waves, are composed of many different waveforms. These are described in the number of cycles per second or *hertz*. A complex mathematic formula termed the Fourier analysis of the complex waveform on the monitor system can reduce it to its individual components. A stereo system may be able to accurately reproduce sound waves from 10 to 20,000 hertz. Accurate reproduction of a biologic signal requires a system that can faithfully reproduce frequencies up to 20 hertz. If the cardiac rate is markedly elevated, perhaps to 180 per minute, however, then 3 pressure signals will be generated in each second and the system must be capable of reproducing frequencies up to 60 hertz. If the system's frequency response is inadequate, the displayed pressure on the monitor will actually be lower than the true pressure generated. This is because the highest frequencies will not be reproduced. This can be illustrated in a simple fashion using only 1- and 2-hertz signals (Figure 2.3). The pressure waveform in this illustration is composed of the sum of 1- and 2-hertz signals. If the monitor can respond to 2 hertz, the true pressure will be displayed. If its frequency response is limited to 1 hertz, it can only display that portion of the curve which is produced by a 1-hertz signal (Figure 2.4). Note that the waveform in Figure 2.3 is displayed as a 2.5 pressure value. The true pressure, comprised of 1- and 2-hertz signals, is actually 2.5. If the monitor can only respond to a 1-hertz signal, the displayed pressure will, therefore, be 2 as in Figure 2.4. Note, too, that a tracing composed of 2 signals has a steeper slope. The clinical implications, therefore, are that a monitor with an inadequate frequency response will display a pressure below the true physiologic signal. This will be found most frequently when heart rates are rapid and the waveform is particularly steep, that is, in a rigid cardiovascular system—elderly patients with hypertension and arteriosclerosis.

The connections between the patient and the transducer influence the frequency response curve. The fluid filled system has a "natural frequency." When the vibrations in the system approach the natural frequency, there is a significant increment in the amplitude of the power signal. This may sound

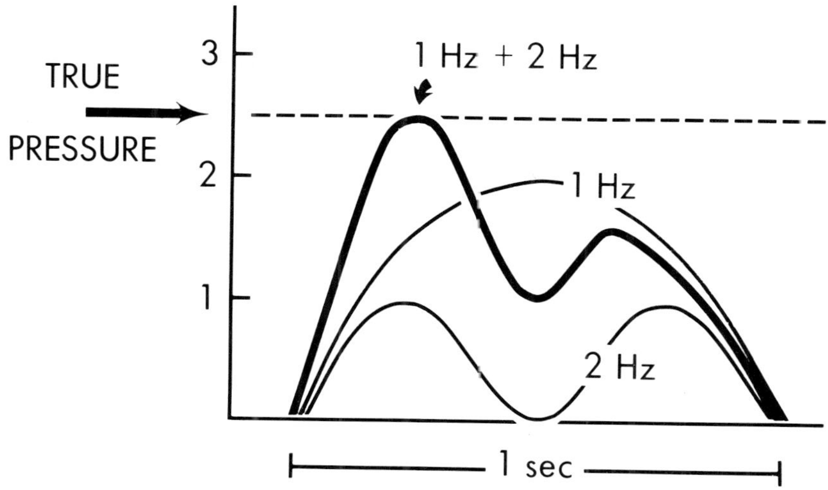

Figure 2.3. Illustration of the waveform produced by 1- and 2-hertz signals. Note that the highest portion of the wave occurs when the individual components are both at peaks.

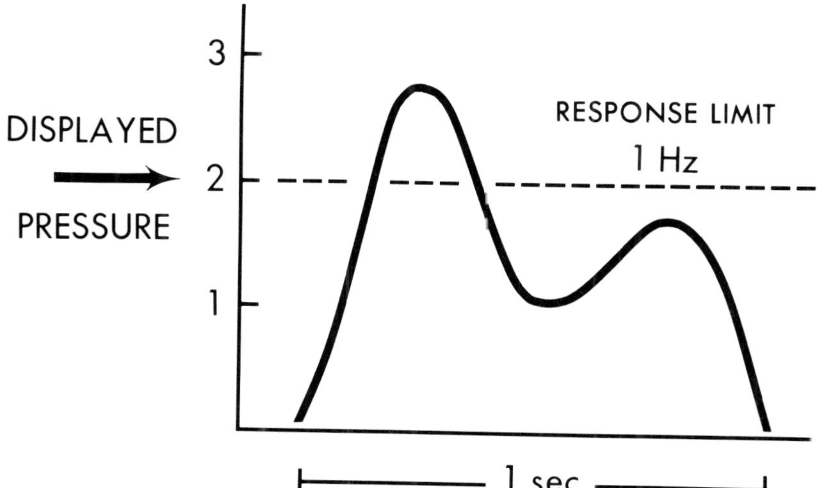

Figure 2.4. Representation of the signal displayed on a monitor capable of responding only to a 1-hertz signal. The highest point cannot be displayed because it represents addition of the 2-hertz signal.

confusing but a simple home experiment will illustrate the physical principle. If one should take an ordinary water glass, wet its lip and rapidly circle the lip with the fingertip, no sound would be produced. If one uses a fine crystal water glass, a ringing sound will be evident. In the crystal, the natural frequency has been reached, amplifying the vibrations to the point at which they become audible. One of the major determinants of natural frequency of a monitoring system is the length of the tubing connecting the catheter to the transducer (Figure 2.5). As the length of the tubing increases, the natural frequency decreases. Thus, an excessive length of tubing will make the natural frequency of the system occur in the physiologic range. The resulting amplification created by the over response of the amplifier circuits causes the displayed pressure to exceed the true physiologic signal. The overall natural frequency relationships are displayed in Figure 2.6. As long as the natural frequency occurs outside the range necessary to faithfully reproduce the biologic signal, 20 hertz, the monitor reading will display the correct blood pressure. If an excessively long piece of connecting tubing is used, however, the system response curve is shifted to the left so that, at 20 hertz, there is already over response or "ringing" in the system. The monitor reading in this situation would overestimate blood pressure because of the amplification in the connecting tubing. This potential must be considered in monitoring the pulmonary system and the length of tubing limited to 4 feet or less.

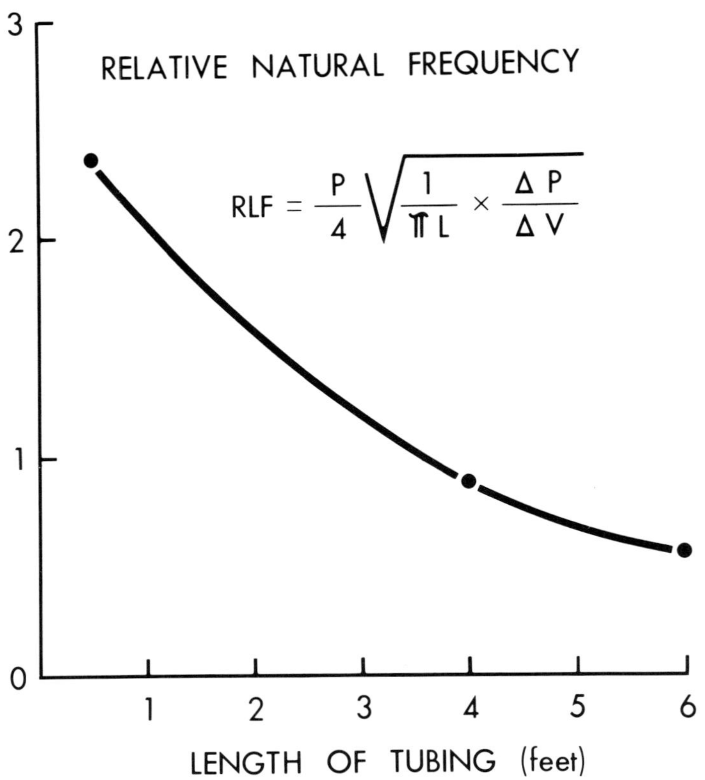

Figure 2.5. Relative natural frequency as a function of catheter length. Note that longer catheter lengths will result in amplification of the signal due to "ringing" in the system.

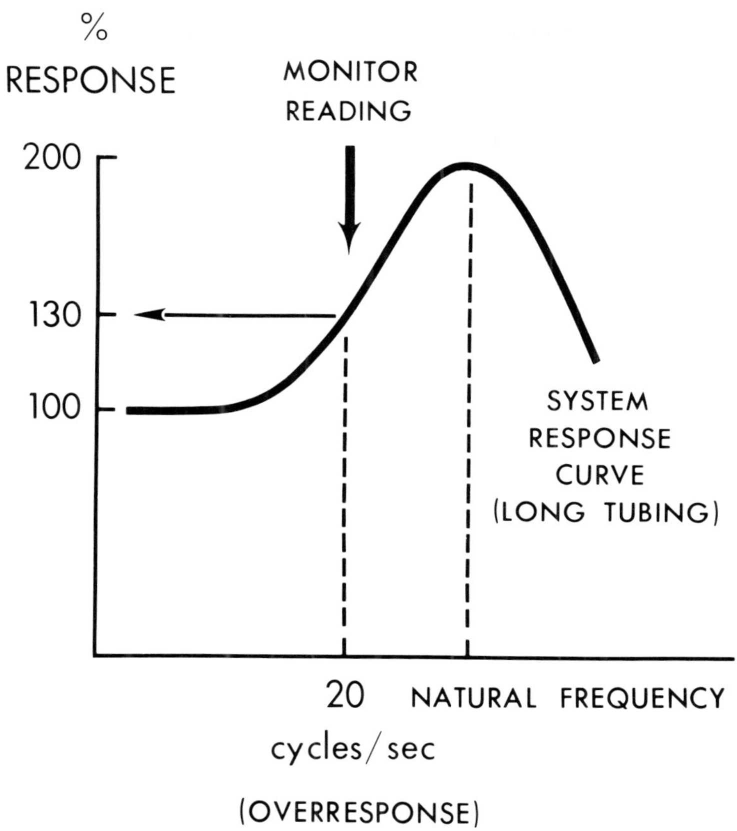

Figure 2.6. If amplification of the signal occurs in the range necessary for accurate representation of the biologic signal, an overestimation of the pressure will be displayed on the monitor.

The third consideration is that of "damping." Damping represents loss of physiologic signal in the transmission system. The creation of the electrical signal depends upon the motion of the diaphragm of the transducer. If some of the physical motion is lost prior to its impact on the transducer membrane, the electrical signal will be diminished because the total physiologic pressure signal has not been applied. If compliant, that is, soft plastic tubing, is utilized to connect the catheter to the transducer, some of the to and fro motion will be lost in expanding the plastic tubing. We use this principle when palpating a peripheral pulse to detect a similar dispersion of physical energy into the expansion of the arterial wall. If low compliant tubing is similarly "pulsatile," energy will be lost and there will be an inadequate representation of the original physiologic signal reaching the transducer diaphragm. The most common artifact to result in damping is an air bubble in the circuit. Fluid is noncompressible. Air, on the other hand, is quite compressible (consider a scuba tank, which contains enough air to fill a phone booth). Transmission of the pressure wave through the tubing to the transducer depends on the noncompressible nature of the fluid. In other words, the exact amount of motion in the vascular system is transmitted to the diaphragm of the transducer. If, however, a bubble is introduced into the system, part of the energy of the fluid will compress the air (Figure 2.7) and thus would be lost at the transducer diaphragm. There would be more motion of the fluid column on the patient's side of the air bubble than there will be at the diaphragm. Less movement of the diaphragm produces a less powerful electronic signal and the displayed pressure is, therefore, lessened (Figure 2.8). The effect of damping is extremely important in measuring pulmonary arterial pressures because there are many high-frequency components to the pressure tracing and the overall pressures are considerably lower than systemic pressures. Thus, damping will cause underestimation of the magnitude of the signal and also, in removing the high frequency components, it may make interpretation of the waveform impossible. A large air bubble in a pulmonary artery catheter system may make the pulmonary artery and pulmonary artery occlusion pressure tracings appear virtually indistinguishable.

The last type of error is known as *catheter whip artifact*. This occurs in the pulmonary arterial circulation and will not be found in systemic arterial pressure monitoring. It is the result of the mechanical transmission of the force of the heart during its contraction. This contraction is so powerful that it imparts an acceleration to the catheter sitting within the pulmonary artery. Envision a cowboy attempting to ride a bucking bronco. The horse's fre-

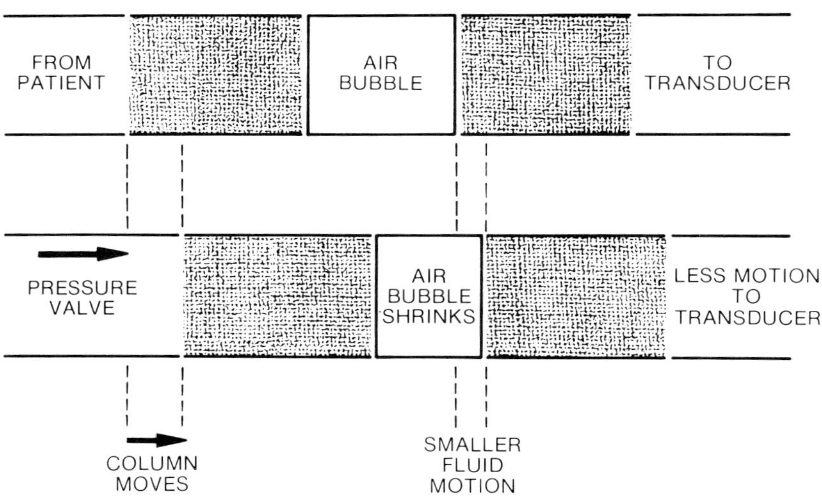

Figure 2.7. The effect of an air bubble in the transmission tubing is depicted. Because the air is compressible, some of the fluid motion generated by pulsatile flow is lost in compressing the air bubble. Thus, the motion which is transmitted to the diaphragm of the transducer is less than that generated by the pulsatile flow.

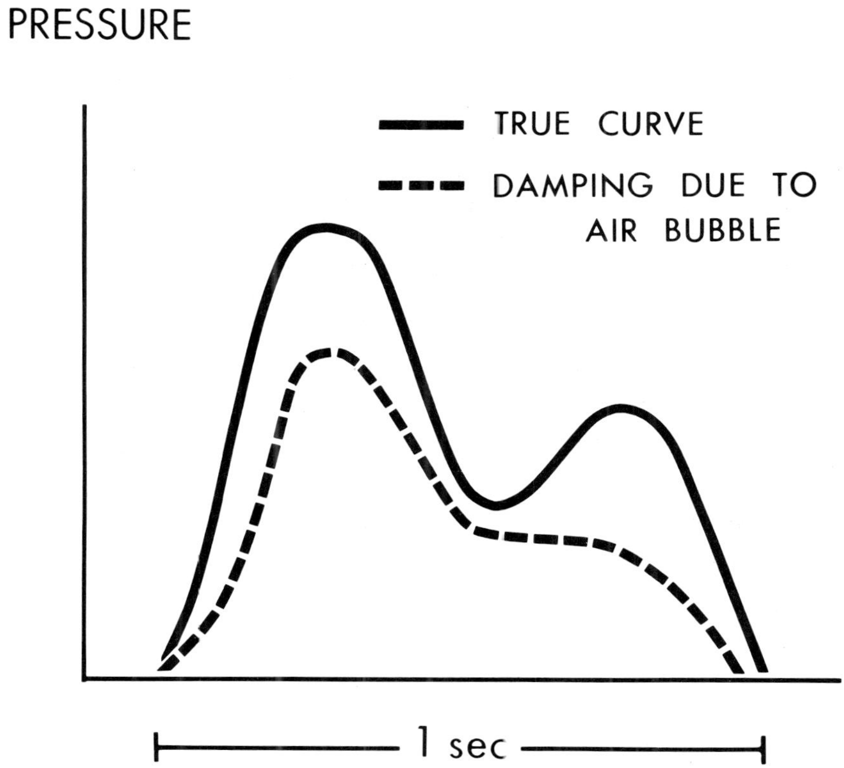

Figure 2.8. Representation of the pressure tracing caused by damping. The true pressure tracing is seen in solid lines representing amplification of the electrical signal emitting from the transducer. If damping has occurred, the signal will be lessened and the resultant pressure tracing will also show lower peak pressures.

netic bucking causes the cowboy's upper body to rock back and forth. The cowboy's head may be considered analogous to the tip of the pulmonary artery catheter. This is a very high-frequency artifact and can be handled effectively by incorporating a filter into the system much as static can be filtered out of a stereo record using a "high frequency" filter.

A practical bedside approach to pressure monitoring has been devised which recognizes these electronic considerations, and yet, attempts to safeguard the equipment. The variable resistance in the transducer diaphragm is extremely delicate. Placing the transducer directly at the patient's bedside subjects it to damage in a busy intensive care unit. We have found that permanently positioning the transducer on the wall behind the bed can reduce breakage of these delicate instruments. The connecting tubing in this position must not be longer than four feet. Finally, accurate calibration of the transducer monitor system must be performed in order to verify that a known pressure signal is accurately displayed.

B. Calibration

Introducing a zero reference point and creating an electrical signal to represent a known pressure are termed *balancing* and *calibrating*. The zero reference signal is usually chosen to be the midpoint of the cardiac chambers. Although it is often suggested that the diaphragm of the transducer be adjusted to this level and atmospheric pressure introduced by opening a stopcock on the transducer dome, this is not necessary or desirable. Remember, it is desirable to leave the transducer in a stationary position to avoid damage to this delicate instrument. It is necessary to introduce an atmospheric signal at the proper level but this can be easily accomplished by assembling the entire system, filling it with fluid, closing the transducer completely and using the unconnected tip of the transmission tubing as the reference point. This can easily be approximated to the appropriate position on the patient's chest wall and introducing this signal by adjusting the zero reference control on the monitor. This has the additional advantage of eliminating the possibility of introducing air bubbles into the transducer dome and minimizes the risks of infection by insuring that the fluid filled system is opened only at the end of the transmission tubing, which can be easily sterilized. The secured and stationary transducer need never be moved to compensate for changes in the patient's position or the height of the bed. It is only necessary to rebalance by disconnecting the end of the transmission tubing and adjusting it to the proper level.

Calibration of the monitor requires introduction of a known pressure signal. This can be done in one of two ways: internal or external calibration. Internal calibration is available on all monitors. It involves activation of the calibration control which introduces an electrical signal to the monitor which corresponds to the desired calibration pressure. This form of calibration can be considered to represent the introduction of electrical signal into the amplifier "as if" that calibration pressure had been applied to the transducer itself. Although the transducers are supposed to be accurate to within ±5%, in practice we have found that this accuracy is rarely achieved if transducers are used for a long period of time in a busy intensive care unit. We tested 16 transducers and found that their accuracy was ±27% (2). Obviously, this exceeds the variability that can be permitted and, therefore, the electronic reference signal may introduce artifact if a transducer with wide variance is used.

Accordingly, a simple external calibration system which, in fact, tests the transmission tubing, transducer, and monitor seems more desirable because it should be more accurate. Using this approach, a column of water equivalent to 20 mm Hg pressure is externally applied to the transducer. Because mercury weighs approximately 13.4 times as much as water, this would require introduction of a water column 26.8 cm (268 mm H_2O). This can be readily accomplished using an IV pole as a calibration tool. An alligator clip is fastened to the zero point (Figure 2.9) and the second clip is fastened at a measured distance of 26.8 cm above the zero reference point. The free end of the transmission tubing is attached to the zero clip. The monitor is then adjusted or balanced to this zero level. The end of the tubing is then elevated to the 26.8 cm or 20 mm Hg (Figure 2.10) reference point and the gain or calibration control is adjusted so that 20 mm Hg are displayed on the monitor. In this system, an actual physical signal representing 20 mm Hg is applied to the transducer diaphragm. The free end of the

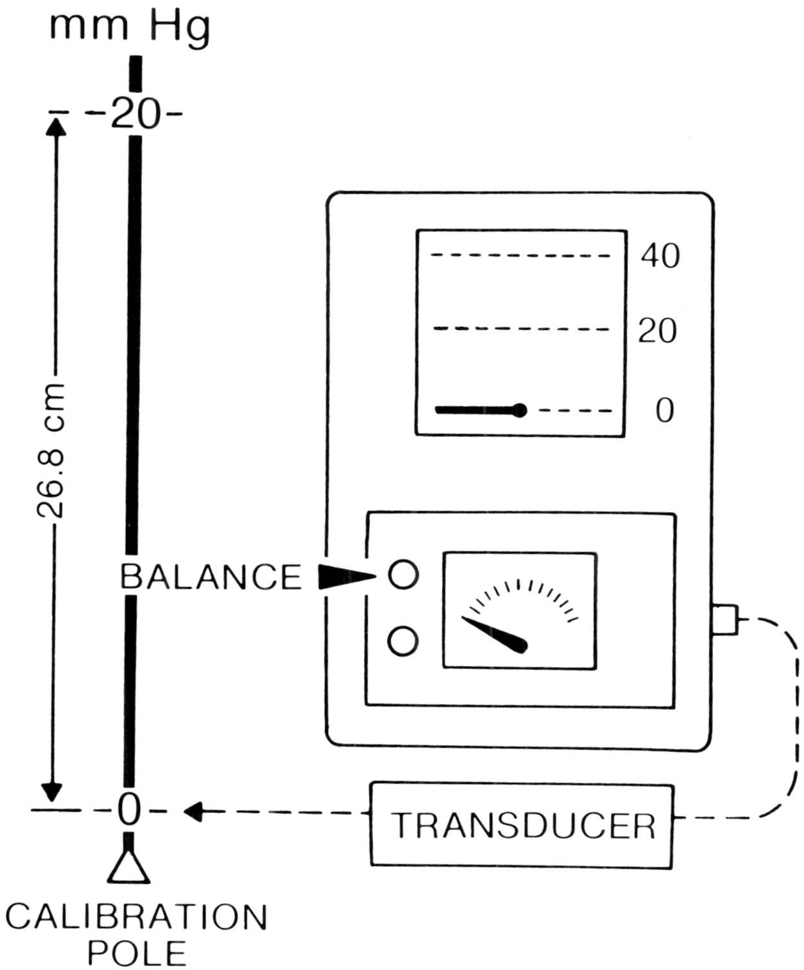

Figure 2.9. External calibration using the introduction of a known signal. The first step is to attach the end of the pressure tubing to the 0 point on the calibration pole. The monitor itself is then adjusted so that this 0 reference pressure is displayed.

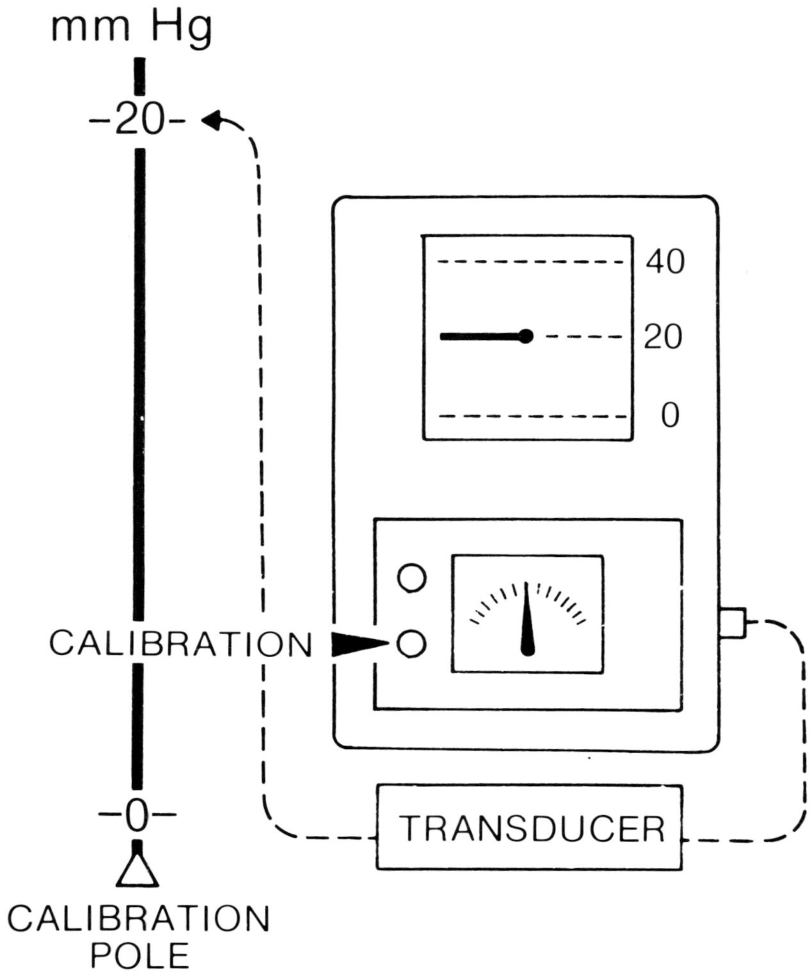

Figure 2.10. Introduction of the actual pressure signal. The end of the tubing is then elevated to a preselected point corresponding to 20 mm Hg (26.8 cm above the 0 reference point). A monitor is then adjusted to reflect this signal.

tubing is then placed at the appropriate location on the patient's chest wall and a zero reference signal—or rebalancing—activated. This process seems easily understandable and, in practice, has been repetitively performed by nurses and technicians with great reliability.

C. Catheter Design

The initial flow-directed pulmonary artery catheter introduced into clinical practice contained two lumens (3). One served for transmission of the pressure signal and aspiration of samples from the pulmonary artery and the second was used to inflate a 1-ml latex balloon positioned proximal to the pulmonary artery catheter tip. After the catheter had been introduced into the central venous circulation, the balloon was inflated and advanced utilizing pressure monitoring through the cardiac chambers until it reached a position in which the balloon totally occluded the pulmonary artery. At this point the character of the tracing changed and assumed characteristics similar to a left atrial pressure tracing. This was termed pulmonary capillary wedge (PCW), pulmonary artery occlusion pressure (PAO), or pulmonary artery wedge pressure (PWP). The initial catheter was a soft and pliable 5 French catheter. A number of additional features have been added to serve special purposes, and others are under development at this time. The most commonly employed catheter today is a 4-lumen, 7 French catheter incorporating a thermistor positioned approximately 5-6 centimeters proximal to the tip of the pulmonary artery catheter and an additional port which is intended to permit pressure monitoring and blood sampling from the right atrium. The 4-lumen catheter thus permits: 1) monitoring of pulmonary artery pressure (distal lumen, balloon deflated); 2) monitoring pulmonary artery occlusion pressure (distal lumen, balloon inflated), 3) right atrial pressure monitoring (proximal lumen); 4) cardiac output by the thermodilution method (thermistor connected to external cardiac output computer); 5) sampling true mixed venous blood (sample aspirated through distal lumen, balloon deflated); 6) sampling right atrial blood (sample aspirated through proximal lumen).

The 7 French catheters are somewhat stiffer than the 5 French models; this facilitates passage through the heart but may also cause the catheter tip to impinge upon the intraventricular septum and promote arrhythmias. The balloon has been designed so that, when properly inflated to 1.5 ml, the tip of the catheter itself is recessed into the balloon. In this fashion, the soft latex balloon rather than the stiff catheter tip will touch the intraventricular septum.

Other catheters are available for use in pediatric patients. Some catheters are 7 French in diameter but have the proximal (right atrial) port positioned 15-20 cm from the distal port. In the catheters used in adults, the proximal port is usually positioned 30 cm proximal to the tip of the catheter. Currently available catheters are catalogued in Table 2.1.

Newer catheters incorporate a fifth lumen containing fiberoptic bundles which can be used to measure mixed venous saturation when connected to the appropriate external instrument. In periods of constant oxygen consumption, mixed venous saturation will vary inversely to cardiac output permitting continuous estimation of changes in cardiac output. In conditions of changing oxygen consumptions, mixed venous saturation and cardiac output may both vary independently, and this information, when combined with thermal dilution cardiac output measurement, may afford insight

Table 2.1 Flow directed catheters

Type	Size (French)	Proximal port (cm)	Thermistor	Other features
Double lumen	5	0	0	0
	6	0	0	0
	7	0	0	0
Triple lumen	7	30	0	0
	7	20	0	0
Pediatric double	4	0	0	0
	5	0	0	0
	5	0	0	Angiography
Pulmonary angiography	7	0	0	0
	8	0	0	0
Bipolar pacing	5	0	0	0
Thermodilution	7	30	+	0
	5	20	+	Pediatric balloon tip
	2.5	0	+	No balloon
	8	30	+	Oximeter connection
	7	30	+	Heparin bonded
	7	30	+	Extra lumen or pacing
	7	30	+	Extra right atrial port

into these changes in overall oxygen consumption. Resuscitation from low flow states and the development of systemic sepsis represent conditions in which both oxygen consumption and mixed venous saturation may vary simultaneously because of changes in total body oxygen consumption.

Other catheters incorporate electrodes that can be used to monitor intracavitary electrocardiograms in both the atria and ventricles. In some instances, these can be used for electrical pacing of the cardiac rate.

The cost of catheters with electrodes are substantially greater than the usual 7 French thermodilution catheter. An additional lumen which terminates in the region of the right ventricle would permit the introduction of an electrode for intracavitary electrocardiogram or pacing if the situation warranted. Thus, the pacing capability would be available, but the cost would not be absorbed by every patient requiring pulmonary artery catheterization for monitoring of hemodynamic parameters. Additionally, this fifth lumen could be used for fluid infusion and perhaps obviate the necessity of an additional central venous catheter.

Another new catheter has a fifth lumen designed to end in the right atrium which can be used for fluid infusions. This can eliminate the necessity to interrupt vasoactive infusions during cardiac output determinations.

Most pulmonary artery catheters in current use are constructed of materials that can be thrombogenic. It is possible that these catheters can become the site of intravascular clot formation. This might result in superior vena caval obstruction or pulmonary emboli. Newer catheters are under clinical evaluation which bond heparin to the catheter in an attempt to minimize this thrombogenic potential.

D. Standardization of Insertion

In addition to providing an accurate monitoring system, standardization of the components used in catheter insertion may be able to diminish the risks of insertion and maintenance of the invasive monitoring technique (4). Accordingly, it seems advisable to collect all necessary components in a prepackaged sterile kit. This is especially important in units in which invasive monitoring is initiated by house officers or residents who only spend a brief period of time on the rotation. They cannot be expected to have investigated the reliability of all components. Ready availability of acceptable components makes it easier to use the kit provided than to gather the necessary paraphernalia in a haphazard manner. Thus, experimentation is diminished and standardization insures the utilization of proper components in a simpler manner, particularly useful in an emergency situation. The external system should be standardized as well. Patency of the pressure monitoring system had been a problem until the introduction of pressure-driven, continuous, low-flow infusion systems. Our own preference is to use a spring-loaded pressure device, such as the Tycos pressure infuser, because the inflatable bags seldom maintain constant pressure after they have been in use for several months. If the driving pressure falls below the recommended 300 mm Hg, the constant infusion device no longer functions and the risk of clotting and loss of the invasive monitoring tool is greatly increased. This may be of greater significance in arterial catheters, but standardization of all procedures is more likely to result in consistent performance. Therefore, the same type of device is recommended for pulmonary artery catheterization. Normal saline solution containing 5,000 units of Heparin per 500 ml can be used as the "flush solution." Sodium administration is minimal because the constant flow device limits infusion to approximately 72 ml per 24 hours. Solutions containing dextrose are less desirable because the possibility of allowing bacterial growth is enhanced. A disposable dome for the transducer eliminates the necessity for gas sterilization of this delicate instrument and allows the system to be changed quickly and safely. Although the use of a fluid interface between the transducer diaphragm and the disposable dome has been incriminated as a source of bacterial contamination, we have not found that a similar risk is incurred if no fluid interface is provided. The frequency response of the system without fluid is sufficiently accurate for clinical measurement. On the other hand, in order to preserve the biologic signal, only low-compliant, rigid pressure tubing should be used to connect the catheter to the transducer assembly. We have not found it necessary to display both pulmonary artery and central venous pressure tracings continuously. Rather, intermittent observation and recording of measurements is satisfactory and, additionally, provides an extra access port for infusions. Accordingly, we use a double low-compliant tubing attached to a stopcock mounted on the continuous infusion device. Each end of the pressure tubing is connected via a double stopcock to the proximal and distal ports of the pulmonary artery catheter. Continuous pressure monitoring of the pulmonary artery can be maintained and fluid infusions given through the central venous port. When central venous pressure measurements are necessary, the double stopcock is turned to its pressure tubing and the integral stopcock in the pressure monitoring system reversed to reveal the central venous pressure tracing. Additionally, this requires dedication of only a single pressure channel on the monitor and may permit adequate hemodynamic monitoring using a single three-channel monitor which incorporates electrocardiogram, arterial pressure, and a single pressure channel for the pulmonary artery catheter. The disposable dome, continuous infusion device, and double low-compliant pressure tubing assembly have been combined into commercially available kits by Gould-Statham and Sorenson. These kits have the additional advantage of being preassembled and having welded connections. Thus, accidental disconnection and contamination are minimized, and considerable time is saved in assembling the external pressure monitoring system. The assembled components are displayed in Figure 2.11.

The prepackaged kit containing the components for catheter insertion contains an outer package with materials for preparing the site and completing the dressing, as well as an inner package containing all the sterile components themselves. Table 2.2 lists the contents of the kit currently in use in the Surgical Intensive Care Unit at the University of Miami/Jackson Memorial Medical Center. This kit requires only the addition of the pulmonary artery catheter itself and a device for percutaneous introduction. The rationale for skin preparation and dressing are described in the following discussion.

II. INSERTION TECHNIQUE

A. Preparation of the Insertion Field

Although the operator is usually concerned with technical complications during insertion, clearly, the most important risk of invasive catheterization is sepsis (5). Careful protocols for insertion and maintenance of hyperalimentation catheters have minimized this risk in this technique, but because of the frequent "breaks" necessary to properly utilize pulmonary artery catheterization, this risk is considerably higher. Principles established for parenteral hyperalimentation which must be compromised need to be examined in terms of the reasons deemed necessary and safeguards that can be em-

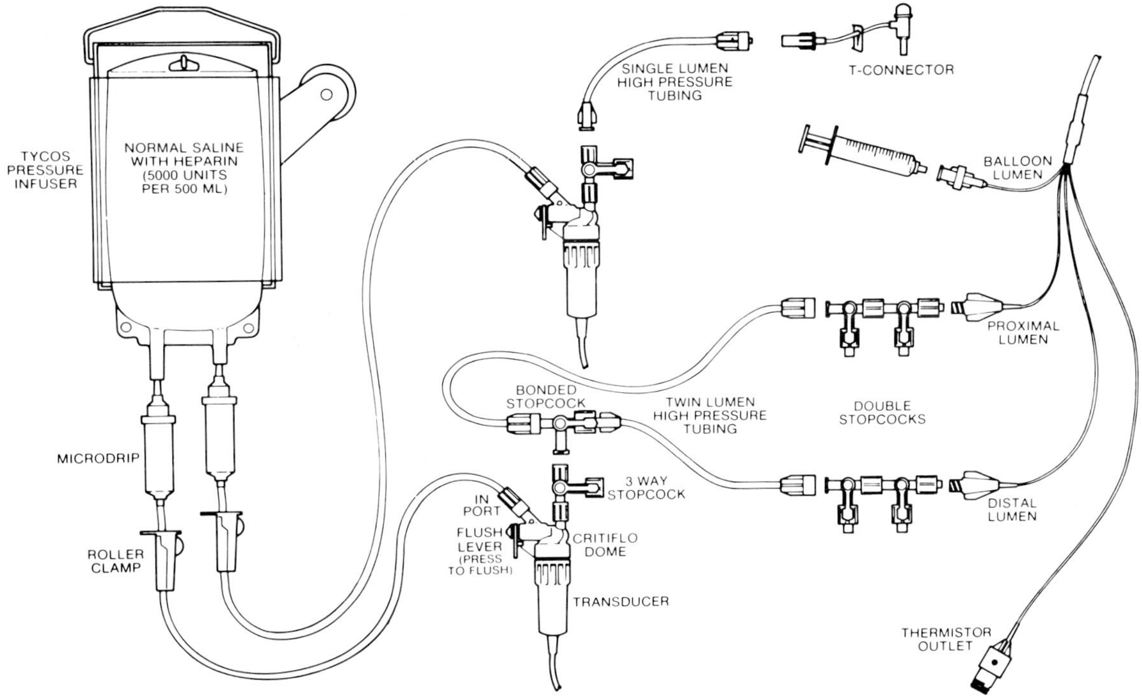

Figure 2.11. External components of pressure monitoring system. A single pressure infuser can be used to power the infusion devices in both arterial and pulmonary artery catheters. The use of a double stopcock enables one transducer to serve both the proximal and distal lumens of the pulmonary artery catheter. Additional components are identified in the drawing and described in the text.

Table 2.2 Prepackaged kit components for catheter insertion

PA Catheter Insertion Kit	
Outer package	1 Sterile sheet 1 Pair sterile gloves, size 7½ 4 Masks 2 Tape, elastoplast (Beiersdorf) patch 4 × 7 1 Roll adhesive tape, 2 inch 1 Roll clear, waterproof tape, 2 inch 1 Betadine ointment 1 Betadine solution
Inner package	1 Scissor, reusable 3 Forceps, reusable 10 Sponges, plain, gauge, 4 × 4 2 Medicine glasses, reusable 3 Towels 1 Scalpel #11 1 Syringe, 10 ml, *non* Luer-Lock 2 Syringes, 3 ml, with 22 gauge 1½ inch needle, *non* Luer-Lock 2 Needles, 18 gauge, 1½ inch 1 Needle, 25 gauge, ⅝ inch

ployed. For instance, a catheter used for parenteral hyperalimentation should not serve as a conduit for administration of medications, other infusions, or for the aspiration of blood samples. Complete monitoring via a pulmonary artery catheter requires frequent injections of iced solution for determination of cardiac output, aspiration of true mixed venous samples from the pulmonary artery lumen, and the use of one or both lumens for the infusion of vasoactive substances or fluid infusions. Although a hyperalimentation catheter should not be manipulated, maintaining the tip of the pulmonary artery catheter in proper position for obtaining wedge pressure often will require subsequent manipulation to reestablish this position. The creation of a proper sterile field and appropriate preparation of the skin are then extremely important in minimizing the risks of invasive sepsis caused by manipulation of the catheter and ordinary use of the monitoring functions. A brief description of our procedure and goals may serve to illustrate a reasonable compromise between ideals and necessities. The patient should be positioned so that the proposed insertion site is easily accessible and free from extraneous equipment such as ventilator tubings, other IV tubings, electrocardiographic leads and other dressings. It is important to secure all of the extraneous equipment before initial skin preparation and creation of the sterile field to avoid subsequent contamination should these extraneous devices "drift" into the field. All personnel at the bedside should wear surgical masks (including an extubated patient) to minimize bacterial contamination from mouth and nasal flora. We have not advocated surgical gowns, similar to procedures for inserting central venous pressure (CVP) or hyperalimentation catheters. One might feel safer if a gown were employed, however, particularly if one is unfamiliar with the equipment or procedure, to safeguard against accidental breaks in technique. The outer wrapper of the insertion kit should be removed and the operator, wearing sterile gloves, should open the sterile inner package. The equipment should be arranged to accommodate additional equipment and to accept the solutions for skin preparation. These include acetone used to defat the skin and remove any traces of adhesive tape, aqueous iodophor solution for its antimicrobial effect, and sterile saline to remove the iodophor solution at the end of the insertion procedure. Acetone should be applied in a circular motion starting at the proposed insertion site from a saturated gauze sponge held in a hemostat. An area of 20-30 cm in diameter should be included. A second application follows. Using this same circular motion, the area should be cleansed three separate times with the iodophor solution. The iodophor solution must be left in contact with the skin surface for at least 2 minutes to insure its antimicrobial action before the actual procedure of insertion commences. The area should be isolated using sterile towels to provide approximately a 20-cm area to aid in establishing landmarks and actual manipulation of the skin. A sterile sheet should be spread from the patient's chest to his feet in order to provide an adequate working area for the pulmonary artery catheter and its connections. It is important to create a large sterile working area because accidental contamination is much more likely if only a small sterile working area is created with the towels.

B. Site Selection—Advantages and Disadvantages

There are many potential routes of access to the right atrium. Whereas the most common determinant seems to be the operator's preference and previous experience, there are particular advantages and disadvantages to be considered for each site. Some of these are related to the technical factors involved in achieving venous access, and others are related to the anticipated duration of catheterization and concomitant diagnoses in an individual patient. In an ideal situation, it would seem that these determinants should be of greater importance than the operator's preference.

Peripheral veins In the initial description of pulmonary artery catheterization in patients who had suffered acute myocardial infarction, catheters were placed via an anticubital vein (3). A "cutdown" or surgical exposure of the vein was often employed. This route and method was familiar to cardiologists, experienced in the cardiac catheterization laboratory; however, it has certain disadvantages in long-term invasive catheterization. These include stasis in the vein used for catheterization, promoting phlebitis; a greater risk of infection in a cutdown site than the percutaneous approach; difficulty in attaining access to the central circulation (navigating the junction of the peripheral vein and the subclavian vein) using the 7 French thermodilution catheters; and an increased likelihood of migration of the catheter tip during necessary manipulations of the patient's position over the ensuing days. Additionally, patients who have been critically ill for extended periods have often thrombosed veins in both antecubital fossae so that they cannot be used for access. The brachial vein which lies beneath the superficial fascia and accompanies the brachial artery may be used in these cases. However, this vein may not be large enough to accept the 7 French catheter. This technique is still useful in patients who have developed coagulopathies. Direct percutaneous access to the larger central veins may be hazardous because the risk of bleeding from inadvertent arterial puncture or laceration of the central vein outweighs the convenience of this more routine approach. Peripheral cutdown can be safely attempted in these unique situations.

Another common peripheral vein used for pulmonary artery catheterization is the external jugular vein. It may often be cannulated percutaneously with ease, and a J wire may be employed to navigate the junction of the external jugular with the larger central venous system (6). Because it is still a peripheral vein, however, stasis may occur, increasing the risk of thrombosis and, common to all access sites in the neck, it is more difficult to apply a sterile occlusive dressing for an extended period of time. However, this technique is suitable for short-term invasive monitoring during anesthesia and the initial 24 hours of postoperative management. Patients with relatively normal ventricular function who must undergo coronary artery bypass surgery or major abdominal vascular surgery usually do not require prolonged monitoring. In these cases, an insertion site in the neck may be convenient for the anesthesiologist and practical for the first postoperative day.

Central Veins The internal jugular vein is often selected as the access site in similar circumstances. Access may be attempted through the sternocleidomastoid muscle, between the two heads as it approaches its insertions, or by drawing the muscle belly medially, and directing the needle behind the muscle body. There are many approaches with as many advocates, but I will limit description to a technique which has been developed especially to ensure safety. In Figure 2.12, a diagramatic representation of the relationship between the internal jugular vein and sternocleidomastoid muscle can be visualized. The point for catheter insertion can be determined to be three finger breadths above the clavicle and one centimeter medial to the posterior border of the sternocleidomastoid muscle. The needle is oriented in a direction parallel to the anterior border of the sternocleidomastoid at an angle of 30 degrees above the horizontal. In this fashion, the needle traverses the muscle belly and should enter the lumen of the internal jugular vein at a depth of approximately ½ to 2 cm. There are numerous possible complica-

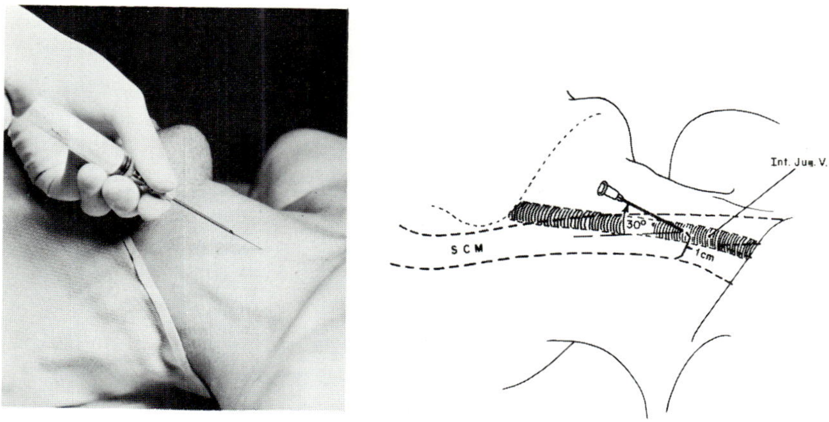

Figure 2.12. Representation of the relationship between the internal jugular vein and the sternocleidomastoid muscle. Note that the spinal needle is used to locate the internal jugular vein and then serves as a guide for subsequent insertion of the larger 14-gauge needle.

tions which can be encountered to secure cannulation of a central vein. These include perforation of an adjacent structure such as the carotid artery, subclavian artery, or cap of the pleura or subsequent perforation of the central vein utilizing the introducer or insertion wire if a modified Seldinger technique is employed. In order to minimize these risks, we have devised the following "safety measures" (7). A #20 or #22 gauge spinal needle is threaded through a 14-gauge needle taken from the catheter assembly system for introduction of a polyethelene CVP catheter. After preparation of the skin and local infiltration with anesthetic solution, both needles are introduced following the guidelines mentioned previously until the internal jugular vein is punctured. The larger needle is then advanced, using the spinal needle as a guide. In this manner, the consequences of inadvertent puncture of an adjacent structure such as a carotid artery will be minimized because the puncture site will be small and manual pressure easily applied to minimize the risk of formation of a significant hematoma. Once the vein has been punctured with the larger needle, a CVP catheter is introduced. I prefer the extra step of cannulation with the plastic catheter to minimize the risk of puncture of the vessel wall if the guidewire is immediately introduced. This technique is recommended for both internal jugular and subclavian cannulation. Others prefer initial puncture with a plastic catheter-over-needle assembly. However, the use of the shorter catheter resulted in puncture of the jugular vein in occasional cases, which led us to employ the longer catheter routinely. After puncture is obtained, the plastic catheter is introduced to serve as a conduit for the subsequent introduction of the guidewire. The risk of subsequent perforation by a guidewire introduced by this technique is real and led us to adopt the intermediate step of introducing the plastic catheter.

When this catheter has been fully introduced and blood aspirated freely from its lumen, one can be reasonably certain that there is no kinking or angulation of the catheter in the lumen of the internal jugular vein. The guidewire can then be more confidently advanced a similar distance. The central venous catheter and its needle can then be removed, leaving the guidewire securely in the lumen of the internal jugular vein. The point of insertion can be enlarged with an 11-blade scalpel and an appropriately sized introducer advanced over the guidewire. It may be necessary to withdraw the CVP catheter 10 cm and cut off the external portion if a short guidewire is used. A long guidewire may obviate this step, but a long guidewire advanced too far has perforated the right atrium and right ventricle. The short guidewire passed through the correctly positioned plastic CVP catheter serves to safeguard against the occasional occurrence of these complications. The operator *must* grasp the portion of catheter near the entry site to prevent it from receding below the skin surface. Subsequent steps are described below.

The disadvantages of the internal jugular approach include difficulty in maintaining a sterile occlusive dressing for extended periods of time and, most commonly, puncture of the common carotid artery. Other, less frequent complications include puncture of the trachea and even the balloon of an endotracheal tube. Obviously, in the latter instance, the operator must have introduced the needle too far and in a medial direction. This complication would be extremely serious during anesthesia or management of a patient with severe hypoxemic respiratory failure. The site is, however, convenient for short-term monitoring, especially if initiated during anesthesia, because the site is convenient and insertion reasonably simple.

Another commonly employed site of venous access is the subclavian vein. This approach has been popularized for intravenous feeding (hyperalimentation) and in the initial descriptions of central venous catheterization for pressure monitoring (8). It has been used extensively in surgical intensive care units for a variety of reasons, including familiarity of approach for the operators and, especially, the ease in maintaining a secure and sterile dressing. It should not be used in patients who have a demonstrated coagulopathy because any complication encountered could be disastrous as direct pressure cannot be applied to the puncture site. Additionally, elderly patients with torturous major arterial vessels may be at higher risk for arterial laceration. In one instance, laceration of a tortuous ascending aorta led to the patient's immediate demise due to massive mediastinal bleeding. These complications can be avoided if parameters of coagulation and chest x-rays are reviewed before attempting subclavian cannulation. Although both a supra and infraclavicular approach to the subclavian vein have been promulgated, the infraclavicular approach seems more frequently utilized. Positioning of the patient is, perhaps, more important in this technique than deciding among the various specific points of insertion. The patient should be placed in a head-down or Trendelenberg position to engorge the vein and increase its pressure; this will increase the likelihood of venous puncture and minimize the risk of air embolism. A roll 4-inches in diameter (sheet or blanket) should be positioned vertically beneath the upper thoracic spine. This will permit the shoulder to be displaced posteriorly and insure that the needle can be introduced horizontally. If the shoulder cannot be displaced posteriorly, it may be impossible to direct the needle in an appropriate direction. The risk of subclavian artery and pleural punctures are increased if the needle is directed posteriorly during its initial introduction. I find it convenient to choose an insertion site at the beginning of the curve as the clavicle begins to rise to meet the sternum. This point permits the needle to slip under the clavicle and is more easily identified than landmarks based upon imaginary division of the clavicle. After infiltration of local anesthetic, I recommend subclavian puncture with a 14-gauge needle taken from a central venous pressure insertion kit. The central venous catheter is then introduced as described in internal jugular puncture. The guidewire is passed through the catheter in a similar manner.

The femoral vein is infrequently used for passage of pulmonary artery catheters. In surgical patients with abdominal sepsis, there are obvious reasons to avoid this approach to maintain sterility of the insertion site. In obese patients, this vein may be hard to locate. Finally, because the risk of deep vein thrombosis and subsequent pulmonary embolism is well recognized, it seems prudent to avoid this site for cannulation with the usual pulmonary artery catheters. If the heparin-bonded catheter can be shown to diminish the risk of thrombosis, this site may be considered again. It will, however, be less satisfactory for long-term monitoring because of the difficulties in maintaining an adequate sterile dressing. This is obviously not an overwhelming contraindication because long-term cannulation of the femoral artery is often used for pressure monitoring in many intensive care units.

The site of insertion can usually be easily identified in patients of normal body habitus. The femoral vein lies immediately medial to the femoral artery. The femoral artery should be identified as it emerges from underneath the inguinal ligament. The insertion site should be approximately 3 cm below this in order to allow the needle to be advanced in a more horizontal fashion. This is in contradistinction to the vertical approach usually recommended for aspiration of femoral artery or femoral venous samples percutaneously. After the vein has been punctured, the technique described for internal jugular and subclavian puncture can then be employed.

I would currently recommend that this approach only be used if the other sites are not available for long-term monitoring. During anesthesia, the femoral site would have the additional disadvantage of being inaccessible to the anesthesiologist during most common surgical procedures. It may, however, be employed if superior vena cava obstruction is present or suspected, and in emergent situations when its ready access may be considered desirable.

Surgical exposure of either the saphenous vein near its junction with the femoral vein and the axillary vein have been necessitated in very rare instances in the author's experience. In desperate circumstances, however, imagination and perseverance should always enable one to find a site of access to the central circulation.

C. Insertion of Final Introducer

There are two methods used to insert the pulmonary artery catheter. The catheter may be directly placed in an exposed vein after it has been isolated surgically, or a conduit may be used to pass the catheter from the skin insertion site to the lumen of the vein. The latter method is used for direct puncture of the large central veins such as the subclavian, internal jugular, or femoral veins. After the CVP catheter has been inserted and blood freely aspirated, a guidewire can be passed to approximately the same distance. This insures that the tip of the guidewire is not blindly introduced and minimizes the risk of perforation. The central venous catheter is then removed, leaving the guidewire in place. The insertion site is enlarged using a #11 scalpel blade. Passage of the introducer (Figure 2.13a) through the subcutaneous tissue can be facilitated if the back of the scalpel blade is aligned with the guidewire and the point advanced 1 to 1½ cm. This will allow the introducer, which is of much larger caliber, to traverse the subcutaneous tissue without requiring a great deal of force or twisting which may tend to damage the introducer and sheath. The introducer assembly usually consists of two portions: a tapered inner section to dilate the tract and venous puncture site, and an outer conduit which will remain in the vein for passage of the pulmonary artery catheter. The dilator is passed through the conduit and both are then advanced over the guidewire. The tapered tip of the dilator should precede the conduit. The conduit itself should be advanced sufficiently so that its tip will remain in the vein cannulated after the guidewire and the dilator are removed. Ordinarily, blood will well out of a properly placed conduit; if this does not occur, a syringe should be attached to the hub of the conduit and manipulations gently performed until a free flow of blood is obtained. A new type of conduit has become commercially available (Arrow, Cordis, USCI, and others) which incorporates a side-arm for continuous fluid infusion (Figure 2.13b). These conduits are left in place after the pulmonary artery catheter has been inserted through the perforated diaphragm on the end of the conduit. A sterile plastic sleeve can be attached to the end of the conduit so that the catheter may be manipulated in a sterile fashion later should its tip become malpositioned. This new device provides an additional central venous port of fluid administration and

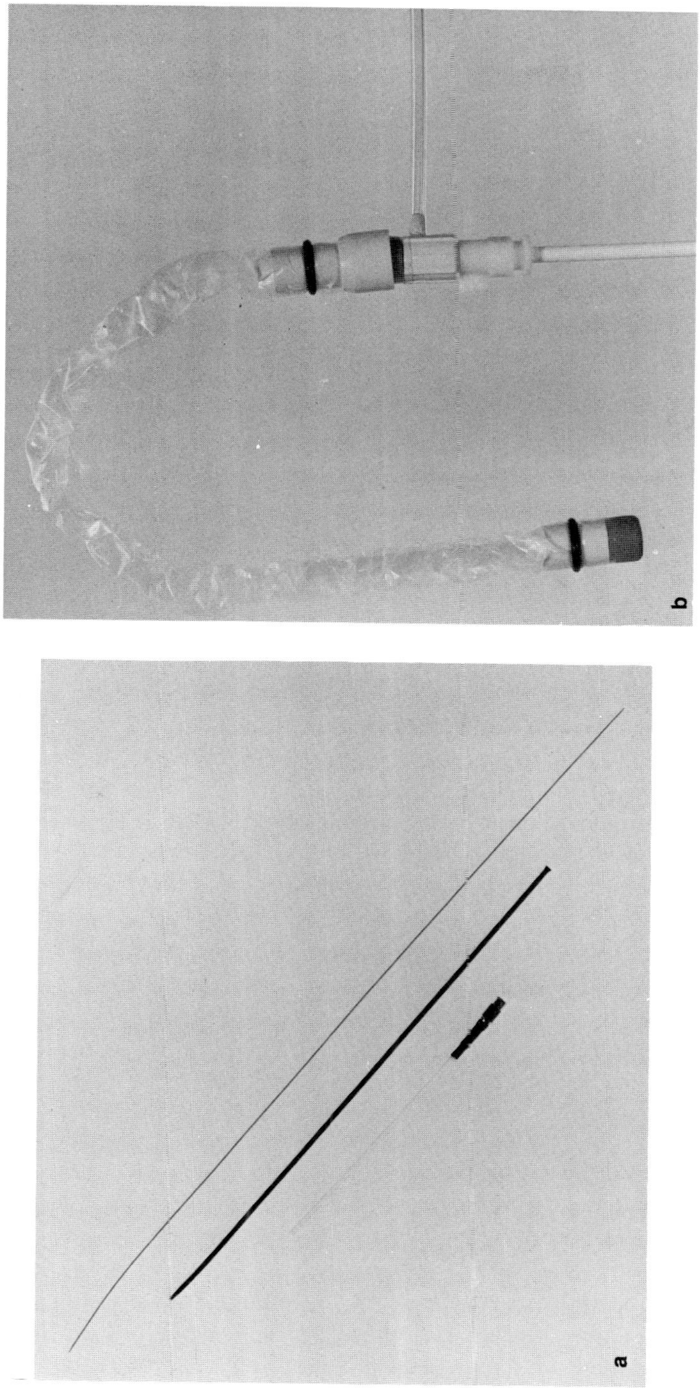

Figure 2.13. Photographs of 2 commonly used introducers. The introducer in *a* is removed once the catheter has been inserted. However, in *b*, a newer introducer is displayed. Not only does the final conduit remain in the place, but this conduit can be used for fluid infused through the side arm.

makes it technically easier to manipulate the catheter at subsequent intervals. There are no data available to judge long-term sterility of the system, although studies are presently in progress. Using this newer type of introducer, initial access to the central circulation can be attained and subsequent insertion of the pulmonary artery catheter can be rapidly accomplished should invasive monitoring become necessary later. The advantages are extremely attractive; however, until data are available to document the sterility of the sheath assembly and perforated diaphragm, it would seem judicious to recommend its use for short-term catheterization.

Once the final conduit is in appropriate position, the catheter itself can be prepared and tested with the help of an assistant. The inner sterile wrapping of the pulmonary artery catheter should be handed to the operator. Once the protective devices have been removed, the distal end containing the balloon, thermistor, and sampling ports should be handed to the assistant. Double stopcocks are attached to the proximal and distal ports, and the lumens are filled by a syringe attached to one of the ports of the stopcock. The low compliance pressure tubing is then attached to the stopcock connected to the distal or pulmonary artery lumen. The central venous pressure or right atrial lumen is similarly filled to test for the patency of the lumen, but the stopcock is then closed off during actual insertion. The balloon is then inflated with 1.5 ml of air and it is inspected for symmetrical inflation and protection of the catheter tip, and left inflated for a period of time to test for leaks. During this time the operator holds the catheter to insure that no contamination occurs. The operator then advances the catheter through the introducer sufficiently so that the catheter tip enters the venous lumen. At this point, the distal lumen is aspirated with a syringe to ensure free flow of blood. The syringe is then used to flush the blood from the catheter, and the stopcock is turned to allow the pressure tracing to be viewed on the monitor. I prefer to have the balloon inflated immediately after the catheter tip is positioned in the lumen of the vein. In internal jugular, subclavian, and femoral cannulations, then, the balloon would be inflated as soon as the catheter tip is introduced. In peripheral cutdowns, the catheter must be advanced sufficiently so that the tip has indeed reached a central vein. This distance is best estimated before insertion of the catheter by holding the catheter over the patient's arm in such a position so that the catheter tip overlies the approximate position of the subclavian vein. The operator notes the mark on the proximal portion of the catheter overlying the antecubital site. I feel that immediate inflation of the balloon maximizes the flow directed properties of the catheter to facilitate reaching the right atrium. Usually, the pressure tracing will reveal characteristics of the catheter's intrathoracic location after the catheter has been advanced approximately 10-15 cm. If the patient is breathing spontaneously, this will be characterized by a sudden deflection corresponding to the inspiratory effort (Figure 2.14a). This is an artifact induced by the sudden diminution in intrathoracic pressure which occurs during inspiration. Alternatively, if the patient is receiving positive pressure ventilation, the tracing will be augmented during the mechanical inspiratory phase. This, again, is the result of an artifact created by intrathoracic pressure (Figure 2.14b). During positive pressure ventilation, airway pressure is considerably above the ambient level and this intrapulmonic pressure is usually transmitted to the intravascular pressure tracings. The catheter should be advanced steadily until a right ventricular tracing is visible, or until 30 cm of the catheter has been introduced from either the internal jugular vein or subclavian position. When an antecubital vein is used, it will require approximately an additional 20 cm (right) or 30 cm (left) before one encounters the right ventricular pressure tracing. If a right ventricular pressure tracing is not visible, there are two possibilities: either the catheter has entered another central vein, that is, the innominate vein or inferior vena cava; or the catheter is curled in the right atrium. If the balloon is immediately inflated after the catheter tip has been positioned in the central vein of insertion, it is unlikely that it can proceed "upstream," because the flow in the other central veins should impede the balloon-tipped catheter from gaining entrance to other central veins. It is not uncommon for the catheter to curl in the right atrium. There are certain obvious physical explanations such as tricuspid stenosis, tricuspid insufficiency, or low-flow states in which the venous flow is so stagnant that flow direction of the catheter tip does not occur. With the balloon still inflated, the catheter should be withdrawn until the balloon impinges upon the introducer tip and the catheter can be withdrawn no further. It should then be advanced again while the operator observes the pressure tracing. Succeeding attempts should vary the rate of insertion and/or rotate the catheter until the right ventricular pressure tracing is vis-

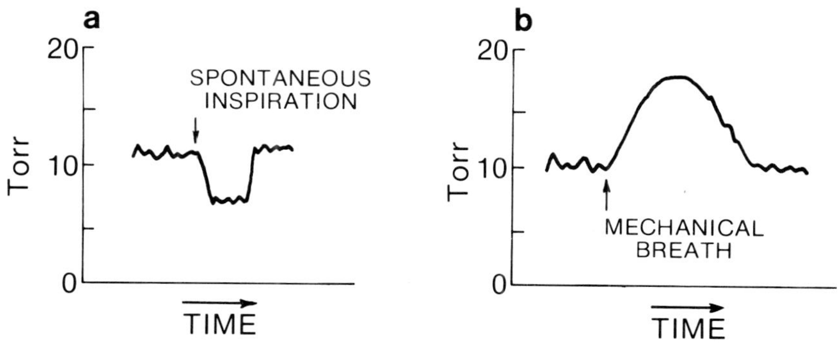

Figure 2.14. Representation of the right atrial pressure tracing in the patient who is breathing spontaneously (a). Note the negative deflection corresponding to the patient's inspiratory effort. Display of a pressure tracing of a patient receiving mechanical ventilation (b). In this instance, the inspiratory effort is followed by a positive deflection of the right atrial pressure tracing.

ible (Figure 2.15). Should this be unsuccessful, further maneuvers are described in a later section. The catheter tip usually traverses the right ventricle after a 10-15 cm length of catheter has been introduced. During this time, ventricular ectopic beats may be induced if the catheter tip impinges upon the ventricular septum. It is always advisable to have the assistant ready to inject an antiarrhythmic, such as Xylocaine, if sustained ventricular beats or multiple ectopic beats are encountered. Withdrawal of the catheter from the right ventricle must be considered if the arrhythmia is deemed sufficiently dangerous or if the Xylocaine administered is ineffective. The right ventricular pressure tracing is characterized by a sharp upstroke, a peak pressure significantly higher than seen in the right atrial tracing and sharp downstroke to the baseline pressure without the presence of a dicrotic notch. The absolute level of the baseline, of course, will depend upon right ventricular end diastolic pressure. Because many patients who are selected for pulmonary artery catheterization have severe disorders of cardiovascular function, it is not uncommon to find this level in excess of 20-25 mm Hg. This would represent some degree of right ventricular failure, but it would be a false assumption to suspect that the pressure could not be "at that level," because the primary reason to use invasive monitoring was because of suspected ventricular dysfunction. It should be obvious that the accuracy of the external transducer monitoring system including accurate calibration and balancing are crucial to the interpretation of abnormal pressure tracings. If the catheter tip is indeed flow directed through the right ventricle, one should see a change in the pressure tracing as the catheter traverses the pulmonary valve. The pressure tracing is altered by the appearance of a dicrotic notch and the diastolic pulmonary artery pressure, which usually is

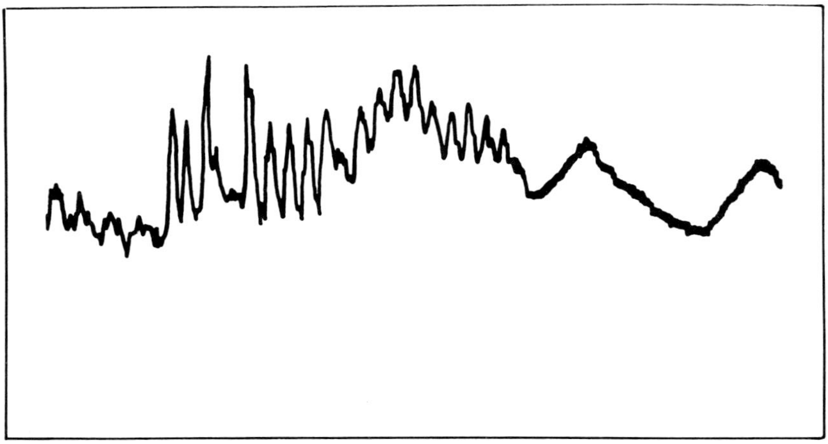

Figure 2.15. A permanent record of a pulmonary artery catheter passed from right atrium to wedge position. Note that the right atrial pressure tracing is followed by right ventricular pressures, pulmonary artery pressures, and, finally, the characteristic wedge pressure tracing.

higher than the right ventricular end diastolic pressure. Certain physiologic disorders result in induced characteristic alterations in the difference between right ventricular and pulmonary artery tracings which will be discussed subsequently. Once the pulmonary artery pressure tracing has been obtained, continual, steady progress of the catheter tip should be maintained until the character of the pressure tracing again changes. This should occur in approximately 5 to 15 cm and is characterized by a low amplitude phasic tracing similar to the right atrial pressure tracing. Obviously, the numerical values of the tracings may often be different, because one of the prime indications for determination of right and left ventricular filling pressures is independence of ventricular function (9). Visual inspection of the pressure tracing is the first criterion used to ascertain correct "wedge" position of the catheter. Occasionally, the wedge tracing may not be sufficiently characteristic to justify this determination. With the balloon still inflated, a specimen can be rapidly aspirated from the pulmonary artery lumen. The initial 2 ml of aspirate should be discarded and a second syringe should be filled with rapidly aspirated blood. The balloon should then be deflated; a second aspiration should be performed extremely slow (1 ml/20 sec) (10). Two ml of this aspirate should be discarded and a second 2-ml aspirate also be obtained at a rate no faster than 1 ml/20 sec. Both specimens should be analyzed in the Blood Gas Laboratory. If the catheter tip is in an appropriate "wedge" position, the sample rapidly aspirated should have a higher oxygen tension than the slow aspirate obtained with the balloon deflated. This differentiation represents "contamination" of the first aspirate with blood which has traversed the pulmonary capillaries, which should have increased oxygen tension. Occasionally the catheter tip may traverse the pulmonary valve, advance into the pulmonary artery, reverse its direction, and come to rest in the papillary muscles of the right ventricle. The damping of the pressure tracing due to the proximity of the catheter tip to the right ventricular musculature may simulate a wedge tracing. However, there will be no difference in the oxygen tensions of the two samples. A chest x-ray should always be taken to ascertain the exact location of the catheter tip. A 1.5-ml inflation volume for the balloon should prevent migration of the catheter tip distally. If the curve of the catheter through the right ventricle is sufficiently gentle, however, it is possible that the catheter tip may still migrate peripherally after the catheter has been secured in correct position. The first step to prevent distal migration can be performed during the insertion itself. After the "correct" position has been obtained, the balloon is deflated to allow the operator to reassess the pressure tracing. The same pulmonary artery pressure tracing should be obtained. The balloon should be reinflated with the expectation that the same wedge tracing will be obtained. This should be done slowly and the amount of air necessary to achieve wedge pressure observed. If it is less than 1.5 ml, the catheter should be withdrawn 5 cm and repositioned. One should attempt to find a wedge position which requires a 1.5-ml inflation volume. Less than 1.25 ml volume should not be considered an adequate final position. This maneuver should be repeated at least two times.

Once the initial position has been verified by repeated inflation and deflation of the balloon, the catheter should be secured in this position. If a removable introducer has been used, the assistant should inflate the balloon until resistance is felt. This should commonly occur at a volume of about 1.5 ml. This is an attempt to "secure" the catheter tip in its proper location while subsequent manipulations are performed. The external position of the catheter is maintained with the balloon thus inflated and the introducer withdrawn over the catheter until its tip is visible. The catheter itself is grasped at the skin level and the introducer moved proximally as far as possible. If an indwelling introducer is used, this step is not necessary and the catheter is secured in its correct position.

As soon as the initial positioning sequence has been completed, the operator must secure the catheter and insure that a proper sterile dressing is applied. The balloon should remain inflated during this final stage to minimize the possibility of migration of the catheter tip. Using the removable introducer, the procedure is as follows: the catheter is immobilized externally, the area surrounding the skin site is cleansed of the iodophor solution with sponges soaked in normal saline. The iodophor solution may cause skin irritation after the occlusive dressing is applied. The area is then dried using sterile gauze squares. An iodophor ointment is then applied to the insertion site and covered with gauze. The antimicrobial iodophor ointment is applied to the catheter insertion site to prevent contamination of the skin entrance site. The catheter itself is *not* sutured in place. A loop of the still sterile catheter is then formed over the first gauze and covered with a second sterile gauze square. The sterile loop of catheter is incorporated in the dressing to limit bacterial contamination, although the catheter itself would be prepared with aqueous iodophor solution if subsequent repositions are required.

The area adjacent to the sterile gauze sponges is then sprayed with tincture of benzoin to form an adhesive surface. The dressing is covered with Elastoplast[R] and a final layer of waterproof tape is applied. The catheter external to the dressing is then immobilized by adhesive tape. Remember to deflate the balloon at this point! The date and time of dressing should be written upon the dressing itself and noted in the patient's record. This will insure that the dressing is maintained properly and changed according to the established protocol. In our Surgical Intensive Care Unit all dressings for invasive catheters are changed each 48 hours. When various catheters have been inserted at different times a routine can be established to change all dressings at the same time; however, this routine time is established by the longest duration of insertion. Thus, if an arterial catheter has been placed 48 hours previously and a pulmonary artery catheter 36 hours previously, both catheters would be redressed at the appropriate time for the arterial catheter. The pulmonary artery catheter dressing might have been left intact for an additional 12 hours, but the convenience for the nurse and reduction in the expensive dressing changing techniques seem to justify redressing the pulmonary artery catheter at the same time.

Except for transient arrhythmias encountered during passage of the catheter, the most frequently encountered complication of invasive monitoring using pulmonary artery catheters is bacteremia (11). Our own experience documented a significant increase in positive blood cultures obtained if pulmonary artery catheterization was continued beyond 72 hours. This incidence dropped dramatically if, in those instances when continued invasive monitoring was deemed necessary, the site of catheterization was changed after 72 hours (12). Although the overall incidence of positive blood cultures was still higher than that encountered in strictly controlled parenteral hyperalimentation, positive cultures were most frequently obtained in patients who had an established sepsis before the initiation of invasive monitoring and the bacteria obtained through the pulmonary artery catheter were usually similar to that cultured from the initial septic source. In patients with established sepsis, it seems prudent to use daily catheter aspirations and peripheral blood cultures to determine if bacteremia develops before the onset of catastrophic clinical illness, that is, septic shock. It also seems prudent to remove any catheter through which a positive blood culture has been aspirated, even if the duration of catheterization has been less than 72 hours. Additional information may be reviewed in the section describing complications.

D. Maintaining an Appropriate Position for Adequate Function

The pulmonary artery catheter serves to provide information with respect to flow (cardiac output), mixed venous oxygen tension, and pressures in the pulmonary circuit and a representation of left atrial pressure. All of these functions are crucially dependent on the correct positioning of the catheter tip. Interpretations of the waveform are subject to error, static x-rays may reveal information which may or may not be interpreted as correct positioning of the catheter, and finally, changes in the cardiovascular status and/or physical positioning of the patient may displace the catheter from its original position. Accordingly, one must be aware of potential errors. One particular catheter position can result in simultaneous and mutually supportive errors in determinations (see below). When the catheter must be repositioned, a method must be constructed to minimize the risk of potential intravascular contamination with bacteria that may have colonized the insertion site or intracutaneous tract of the catheter. The position of the catheter must be assessed by a method relevant to function, because it is impossible to visualize the catheter tip in its final position in the properly sized pulmonary artery.

Errors may result from migration of the catheter tip to a more distal location in the pulmonary artery. The measurement of cardiac output is dependent upon adequate sampling of the injected fluid bolus through the thermistor located 5 cm proximal to the catheter tip. The thermistor should be located in a main pulmonary artery or one of its major subdivisions. Flow around the thermistor will then be representative of total cardiac output because the catheter itself occupies a relatively small portion of the cross-sectional area of the artery in which sampling occurs. If the tip of the catheter migrated peripherally, the thermistor might be located in a much smaller pulmonary artery which either received a less representative portion of total pulmonary artery flow or, because of its small cross-sectional area, created a situation in which the thermistor was closely approximated to the vessel wall. In either of these circumstances, flow surrounding the thermistor itself might not be representative of total pulmonary flow. One might infer that it would sample a lessened flow and, according to the mathematical function of the computer algorithm (see below), would result in the calculation of a higher cardiac output. Unfortunately for the clinician, this position might also create a situation in which careful aspiration of a "true mixed venous specimen" would, because of the low, forward pulmonary arterial flow, result in a mixed sample consisting of true mixed venous blood and blood aspirated from the pulmonary capillaries. This "contaminated" specimen would contain a higher oxygen content. The combination of high cardiac output and high mixed venous oxygen content could be easily considered to represent compensatory mechanisms according to the Fick principle (13). If oxygen consumption was constant and cardiac output did increase, one would expect to find an increase in venous oxygen content reflecting the decreased arterial venous oxygen content difference. A peripherally placed pulmonary artery catheter, then, can result in results that would be compatible with physiologic explanations.

The most common reasons to reposition a pulmonary artery catheter are observation of a continuous PWP tracing (indicating the catheter tip has already migrated to a distal position) or an inability to achieve a satisfactory PWP tracing when the balloon is inflated. Because the former also implies that the methods for ascertaining flow and venous sampling will be in error and the latter eliminates the possibility of accurate determination of left ventricular filling pressure, it is clear that the catheter position must be changed. Using the technique wherein the introducer is removed from central venous access, the following technique for repositioning of the catheter is recommended. An assistant removes the external, nonsterile covering of the "dressing change kit." Similar constraints concerning position and utilization of surgical masks are employed according to the principles outlined previously. The assistant removes the external tape coverings of the insertion site and then suspends the free portion of the pulmonary artery catheter to permit the operator to remove the inner gauze dressings and prepare a sterile field (Figure 2.16). The superficial sterile gauze is removed and the operator grasps the portion of the catheter that has been previously maintained within the sterile dressing. The inner gauze is removed and acetone applied to remove the iodophor ointment and remnants of adhesive tape. This will also serve to defat the skin surrounding the insertion site. Gauze sponges saturated with iodophor solution are then applied to the skin site, surrounding areas, and the protected catheter loop. Because this loop is usually 10-15 cm in length, manipulation of this catheter through the intracutaneous portion should never result in the introduction of any catheter previously exposed outside the occlusive dressing. Although this portion may not be completely sterile before application of the iodophor solution, its protection in the dressing should have insured that it is not grossly contaminated. Preparation of the catheter site and skin areas with an iodophor solution left in contact for 2 minutes should be sufficient to insure sterilization of this portion of the catheter. The operator must maintain a mental differentiation of the function of his extremities: one hand holds the catheter for stabilization during sterilization and the other advances or withdraws the sterilized

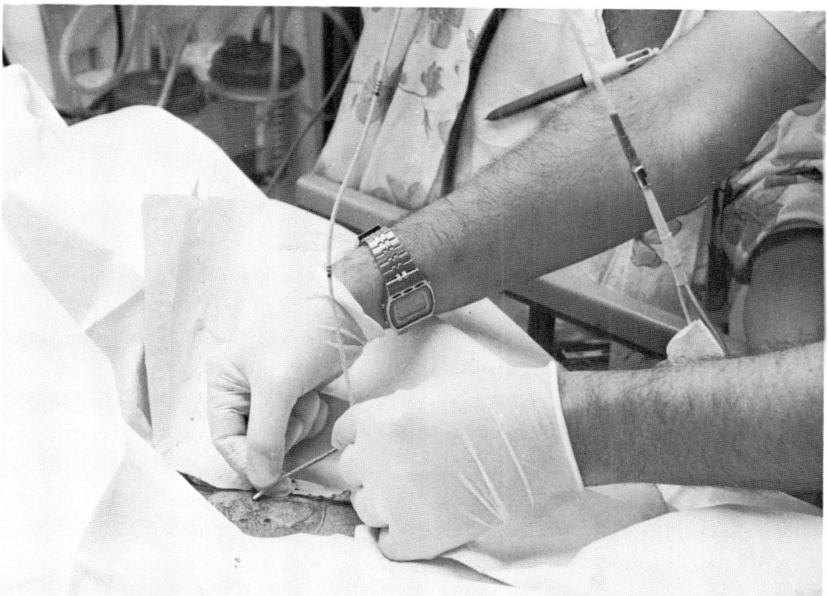

Figure 2.16. Technique for repositioning of pulmonary artery catheter. The assistant suspends the catheter in such a way that the operator can create a new sterile field and coat the exposed portion of the catheter with iodophor solution. Only that portion of the catheter that had been previously contained in the sterile dressing will be manipulated.

portion. After the sterilization procedure has been completed and the area draped with appropriate sterile towels, repositioning can be attempted. If the catheter has been observed to produce only a PWP tracing, it should be withdrawn in 1-cm increments with a sufficient period of observation between each step of the withdrawal process to ascertain if a pulmonary artery tracing can be visualized from the monitor. After a pulmonary artery tracing is again visualized, the operator instructs the assistant to inflate the balloon slowly so that both may observe the onset of the characteristic PWP tracing. At that instant, the assistant should note the volume of air injected into the balloon. If it is less than 1.5 ml, the balloon should be deflated and the withdrawal process continued. Because of the concomitant errors in estimation of cardiac output and mixed venous oxygen saturation, it is necessary to insure that the PWP tracing is only obtained after 1.5 ml of air has been injected. A lesser volume implies that the tip is still in a small pulmonary artery. A greater volume risks potential rupture of the balloon due to an increased inflation pressure. In instances in which the pulmonary artery tracing does not convert to a PWP tracing upon normal inflation of the balloon (1.5 ml), the catheter should be cautiously advanced until the proper tracing is again obtained.

Bedside validation of the position of the catheter tip for determination of cardiac output and aspiration of mixed venous samples can be determined as follows: after a sterile field has been prepared, the operator withdraws the catheter until the pressure tracing again resembles right ventricular pressures. A catheter is advanced 5 cm after the pulmonary artery tracing is obtained. At this point, the thermistor will be in the main pulmonary artery. Because the catheter tip itself is located in the pulmonary artery, a specimen of blood aspirated in this location should represent true mixed venous oxygen tension. Thus, once this position has been obtained, cardiac output should be determined and a specimen aspirated according to the previously mentioned guidelines. The catheter should then be advanced while the observer monitors the pressure tracing until the first appearance of a PWP tracing. The cardiac output and mixed venous sampling should be repeated at this point. Despite the inherent time delay, the catheter should not be fixed and incorporated into a sterile dressing until the results of the two sets of measurements are obtained. A correctly positioned catheter must produce similar results from both positions. One cannot assess changes in the patient's pathophysiology or in response to treatment based on "numbers" created by the invasive monitoring system if the catheter is not properly positioned. This problem is intensified in the era in which the numbers from invasive monitoring are fed into computer systems which calculate "sophisticated values" of cardiovascular function (14). One must always remember the basic principle of computed variables, GI = GO (garbage in = garbage out).

Accurate representations of pulmonary artery pressures, pulmonary artery flows, and pulmonary oxygen tension can be obtained if the operator desires the information and perseveres through technological setbacks. This will be true if the initiative to begin invasive hemodynamic monitoring was based on the desire to replace the uncertainty of clinical judgment with precise characterization of the extant hemodynamics. An inadequately positioned catheter only serves to displace the site of clinical uncertainty from observation of intermediate and inaccurate peripheral observations with unreliable data produced by an inoperative intravascular system. Possible causes and solutions to problems that occur during pulmonary artery catheterization are summarized in Table 2.3.

After the catheter has been correctly repositioned, scrupulous attention must be directed to insure that the new dressing is created according to principles enumerated in relation to the primary dressing. It must also be remembered that each repositioning introduces an additional possibility for bacterial contamination. However, our own data attempting to delineate the risk of intravascular catheterization did not support the idea that repositioning resulted in an increased incidence of bacteremia (12).

If, however, one of the newer introducer systems is utilized wherein the conduit is maintained in the central venous position and the procedures to attach the sterile sheath and other components are carefully observed, it may well be possible to reposition the catheter simply by grasping the catheter through the flexible plastic sheath. It must be reemphasized that, at the present, no comprehensive data have been reported to ascertain that all components of the system remain sterile and that sequential cultures of the external system and subsequent sampling of the blood aspirated through the catheter and peripheral blood have been reported to document the overall safety of this system. Although the principles envisioned seem to be designed in accordance with currently accepted sterile techniques, before this system can be recommended, it will be necessary to ascertain that these manipulations can be performed with reasonable assurance that bacterial contamination has not occurred.

III. PURPOSES OF PULMONARY ARTERY CATHETERIZATION

Three sets of measurements may be obtained using the pulmonary artery catheter: pressures, oxygen tensions (and oxygen contents), and estimations of cardiac output.

A. Pressures Measured

Four pressures have been previously mentioned, pulmonary artery systolic, diastolic, and mean pressure, and PWP. Gradients between observed

Table 2.3. "Trouble shooting" and problem solving

Problem	Cause	Prevention and/or treatment
1. No wave form displayed on oscilloscope	1. Stopcock position incorrect	Correct position
	2. Clot in catheter	Aspirate catheter and irrigate
	3. Loose transducer dome; Air in dome; Defective dome	Irrigate dome and flush out air; Change dome
	4. Transducer not connected properly; Defective transducer	Properly plug-in transducer; Check transducer with mercury manometer; Replace if faulty
	5. Amplifier still on cal, zero or off	Check amplifier
2. Damped pressure recordings	1. Pressure bag not blown up to 300 mm Hg or leaky	Check pressure bag; Replace if necessary
	2. Air in transducer or tubing	Aspirate catheter; Flush air bubbles out of system
	3. Leak in system	Tighten all connections and flush system
	4. Blood clot at distal tip of catheter or blood on transducer	Aspirate blood and flush catheter and/or transducer
	5. Fully clotted catheter (blood is withdrawn and catheter cannot be flushed)	Reaspirate blood; Avoid flushing; Replace catheter if necessary
	6. Kinked tubing or catheter	Inspect tubing and catheter (remove dressing) for kinks; Straighten and splint if necessary
	7. Transducer not open to catheter	Open transducer
	8. Incorrect calibration or gain	Recalibrate and use correct monitor settings
	9. Catheter tip lodged against vessel wall	Ascertain proper position; Reposition catheter if necessary

3. Very low pressures, little difference noted during passage of catheter	1. Damping—As above	As above
	2. Hypovolemia	Verify; treat with volume
4. No right atrial tracing during insertion	1. Catheter curled in SVC or entered other vein	Withdraw catheter with balloon inflated until resistance felt; Readvance
5. No right ventricular tracing	1. Curling in right atrium	Twist catheter; Vary rate of insertion
6. Inability to pass pulmonary valve	1. Curling in right ventricle	Withdraw and readvance; Raise head of bed; Use inotropic agent ($CaCl_2$ or infusion of cathecholamine); Consider fluoroscopy
7. Arrhythmias	1. Catheter tip hits right ventricle	Lidocaine bolus; Check proper balloon volume; Withdraw catheter if arrhythmia persists
8. Persistent difficulty in passage of catheter	1. Unusual anatomic or physiologic changes	Use fluoroscopy
9. Pulmonary artery wave form visible but wedge (PWP) not observed when balloon inflated	1. Catheter tip may not be far enough out in pulmonary artery	Advance catheter
	2. Insufficient amount of air used to inflate balloon	Reinflate balloon with correct volume
	3. Ruptured balloon (no resistance during balloon inflation; Blood aspirated from balloon valve)	Discontinue balloon inflation
10. Continuous PWP wave form	1. Balloon left inflated	Deflate balloon
	2. Catheter tip has advanced too far forward	Reposition patient; If PWP persists, withdraw catheter
	3. Stopcock may be in a closed position	Open stopcock to transducer

Table 2.3. (Continued)

Problem	Cause	Prevention and/or treatment
11. Abnormal PWP or unusual tracing	1. Catheter reversed direction and is in the right ventricle	Withdraw to right atrium and readvance: Obtain chest x-ray to locate tip
	2. Catheter tip against wall	Check for proper balloon volume; Reposition catheter
12. Drastic changes in pressure tracing	1. Altered location of catheter	Check catheter position; Reposition if necessary
	2. Improper calibration or position of transducer	Recalibrate and/or reposition transducer
	3. Measurements taken with patient in different positions	Record pressures with patient in the same position
13. Abnormally low or negative pressure	1. Loose connections	Check connections
	2. Incorrect calibration	Recalibrate correctly
	3. Improper transducer level (higher than atrial position)	Maintain or return patient to same correct position for pressure measurements
	4. Marked respiratory variation	Determine pressure directly from wave form and not from electronic monitor
14. Busy tracing	1. Catheter whip artifact	Check high frequency filter on the monitor; Reposition catheter.
15. Bleeding		
From catheter or tubing	1. Leak in system	Tighten all connections and flush system
From insertion site	2. Improper technique; Vessel trauma	Inspect insertion site; Local pressure and correct fixation

pressures may also be useful. If pulmonary vascular resistance is not elevated, there will be relatively little difference in the observed values for pulmonary artery end-diastolic pressure (PAEDP) and pulmonary capillary wedge pressure. In the absence of right ventricular dysfunction, there may be relatively small differences observed between pulmonary artery end-diastolic pressure and right ventricular end-diastolic pressure. An increase in either of these gradients may be interpreted as inferential evidence suggesting right ventricular dysfunction or elevated pulmonary vascular resistance. In fact, it has been previously reported that the PAEDP and PWP correlate with the degree of abnormality encountered in gas exchange during acute respiratory failure (15). It is also clear that patients suffering chronic obstructive pulmonary disease may develop increased pulmonary vascular resistance resulting in an increase in PAEDP-PWP gradient and evidence of right ventricular dysfunction.

B. Cardiac Output

The technique for measurement of cardiac output incorporated in the thermodilution catheters is extremely simple. Flow or cardiac output is calculated from the Stuart Hamilton formula for indicator dilution (16). This formula has also been used to calculate cardiac output using indocyanine green as the indicator. This method was extremely complex and required sampling of the blood in an external system, calibration of the "cardiogreen" dye in premixed specimens of the patient's blood extracted, and therefore, limited the number of determinations for an individual patient and for an individual unit to, perhaps, 8 or 10 measurements per day. The thermodilution method uses the difference in temperature between the fluid injected and the patient's baseline temperature to represent the amount of "injectate." This method measures the temperature of the injectate, the change in temperature which occurs over time in the pulmonary artery after injection and uses a microprocessor to "solve" the indicator dilution formula. Whereas the initial cardiac output "computers" required the operator to enter the temperature difference and adjust the baseline output of the Wheatstone bridge incorporated to detect the differences in resistance experienced by the thermistor in response to the varying temperature of the blood flow induced by the injectate, the current generation of commercially available equipment performs many of these functions automatically. Unless the operator understands the steps involved, it is possible that the final result may be colored by methodological errors introduced by an unknowing or inexperienced operator. The formula states that flow (cardiac output) equals certain constants multiplied by the amount of injectate divided by the mathematical expression relating the appearance and disappearance of the change in temperature over time. This can be expressed as:

$$CO = \frac{K \times INJ}{\int_{0}^{\infty} \Delta T \, dt}$$

where CO = cardiac output; K = systems constants; INJ = amount of injectate; and ΔT = change in temperature sensed by thermistor. The amount of injectate reflects the volume injected, usually 10 ml, the temperature of the injectate, and the amount of temperature difference "lost" in traversing the catheter from injection port in the external catheter to the port in the central circulation. The temperature difference is now "automatically" calculated *if* the injectate probe is correctly positioned to sample a temperature consistent with the solution actually injected. The central core temperatures are automatically determined by the computer because the thermistor denotes a specific temperature as designated by its electrical resistance. The thermodilution method will be accurate if there is a significant temperature differential between the body temperature and injectate temperature. The simplest technique is to use a "room temperature" injectate. It is more complex to use the originally described 0° C injectate (ice water) technique. However, accurate determination of cardiac output depends upon the amount of injectate that reflects temperature differentiation. Because the error of the method is ±5%, it would seem that the greater injectate, the lesser the potential error of the method would incur. For instance, if the patient's body temperature is 37° and the injectate temperature is 25°, the "amount" of temperature differential is 12°. Cardiovascular analysis may well be necessary in patients whose body temperature is 29° or 30° resulting in a 4° temperature difference. Because the injectate probe cannot be located in the sterile solution which serves as the source of the injectate for cardiac output determination, even a 1° difference in sampling between the actual "room temperature of the injectate solution" and the sample medium of the injectate probe could introduce a 25% error in cardiac output. If a 0° C temperature injectate is used, however, ordinarily there would be a 37° difference in injectate temperature. A 1° error in determination of injectate temperature would, therefore, only cause a 3% error in determination of cardiac output. If the patient's body temperature decreased to 30°, this potential error would be increased to 3.3%. Because of the greater specificity afforded by injection of a larger sample, we have continued to use iced injectates. In order to insure sterility and reproducibility, we have investigated many means of cooling the samples. Our present recommendation is to create an ice bath of large volume and submerge individual containers for each patient. One of the containers is selected to serve as a receptacle for the injectate probe. Individual specimens are withdrawn through a sterile stopcock-and-needle assembly. No cross contamination can occur because each patient's injectate is isolated and all syringes and needles are discarded after a single use. The entire ice bath system has been tested in a clinical simulation. Specimens were aspirated in random fashion, from different containers, and temperature of the injectate was measured using commonly encountered time delays and frequency of injections. Less than 0.2° variation was noted. Sequential and random cultures verified that this method of isolating and cooling injectate samples remains sterile. We only use an injectate container for 24 hours. The 250-ml container contains only sufficient injectate for eight controlled cardiopulmonary investigations (each determination requires three injections of 10 ml). Thus, additional containers of injectate are often required within a 24-hour period.

Again, it may be convenient to examine our methods to insure safety for the patient. Unlabeled sterile containers of the injectate medium (5% dextrose in water) are kept refrigerated to minimize the time necessary to insure that the injectate temperature approaches the selected 0° C level. We have determined that refrigerated containers require submersion in the ice bath for approximately 15-20 minutes before they can be assumed to have been cooled to the desired level. Containers that have not been refrigerated require at least twice that time to reach the same temperature. The probe is placed in a special container for this purpose. Other containers are labeled with name, date, and the time. All containers are changed each morning so that there is no possibility that an individual container will be used for more than 24 hours. Obviously, most containers are used for a shorter period of time. A sterile 18-gauge needle is inserted into a sterilized port of the container. A sterile 3-way stopcock is attached to the hub of the needle. A disposable plastic syringe is attached to the stopcock and a 10-ml volume is repeatedly aspirated and reinjected into the container for 30 seconds. We have previously ascertained that the solution in the syringe achieves equilibrium with the injectate in the iced container within 15 seconds and that this temperature remains constant for at least 30 seconds after termination of the aspiration-reinjection technique. We are thus assured that the injectate in the syringe approximates the temperature of the control measured by the probe for more than a sufficient time to implement the other steps necessary. Because the injection procedure necessitates an additional "break" in sterile technique by requiring the injection of this aspirate through the proximal port of the pulmonary artery catheter, we attempt to use a reasonable technique. The operator must complete a 2-minute handwashing procedure utilizing an effective, hospital-recommended antiseptic solution. He dons sterile gloves and places sterile drapes over the area upon which the exposed ends of the pulmonary artery catheter must be placed. After the injectate has been correctly aspirated from the ice filled containers, the distal or right atrial port connection with the double stopcock is "disconnected" after the fluid and/or pressure monitoring lumens have been blocked by the stopcock positions, and the sterile disposable syringe is inserted directly into the catheter hub. The computer controls are activated and the infusion completed in less than 4 seconds. Operators are trained to time this injection and are audited routinely. Automating the injection systems have been promulgated; however, they introduce additional sources for contamination, breakdowns, and in fact, represent a complex technological solution to a simple problem. The injection should not be automated because the level of ventilatory support, changes in observed pressures relevant to cycling of the ventilator, extraneous movements of the patients, and many other subjective variables can be discerned by an intelligent and educated operator. This more than offsets the slight variability in rate of injection created by manual injection. In fact, the computer algorithms compensate more than adequately for the variations in an injectate time, but no computer algorithms can be created to incorporate the sentient functions of the injector relevant to the critical state of the patient studied. Most cardiac output computers automatically calculate differences between injectate and body temperature (17). One striking human error reflects undue reliance upon the computer calculations. For instance, if a 0° C injectate system is used, its proper constant is entered into the computer by the operator. The computer calculates the actual temperature difference between the patient's observed temperature and that of the probe presumably sampling the injectate temperature. I have personally observed an injectate probe that slipped out of the control container so that the probe was, in fact, recording room temperature. The operator could not understand that the computer calculated the cardiac output to be 25 liters/minute. However, the computer sensed a 12° difference between injectate and room temperature, that is, true room temperature and body temperature, whereas the injectate, in fact, contained 3 times as much "cold." Simply replacing the injectate probe from its accidental location to its correct position in the iced dummy container resulted in an accurate—and physiologic—determination of cardiac output, 8.3 liters/minute. The operator must ascertain that the conditions under which any mechanical device automatically calculates any variable are appropriate.

The computer functions can be summarized. The injectate decreases the temperature of the blood with which it mixes. This change in temperature, which becomes maximal upon completion of the injection and returns to baseline as subsequent blood flow dilutes and carries the injectate into the pulmonary artery, is sensed by the thermistor, a device in which electrical resistance varies in a defined mathematical relationship according to the temperature to which it is exposed. This electrical resistance is incorporated as the variable resistor in a Wheatstone bridge. In earlier cardiac output computers, the resistance of the circuit was adjusted manually so that electrical output of the bridge returned to zero. This function is now automatically provided by the computer which flashes a "ready light" when electrical neutrality is established. Thereafter, any change in temperature "unbalances" the Wheatstone bridge in a similar fashion to that described for pressure transducers. The electrical current in this instance is fed into a potentiometer which calculates the mathematical expression of this change in temperature which is the denominator of the Stuart Hamilton indicator dilution formula. The rest of the computation is simple, the product of the defined injectate temperature and volume is multiplied by the constant previously determined for the catheter system and finally is divided by the output of the potentiometer. Correction factors are incorporated and cardiac output, in liters per minute, is rapidly displayed upon the output device of the computer. The time delay represents the time necessary for the computer to ascertain that the observed temperature decay curve corresponds to the mathematical description of such a curve (an exponential function). Commonly, 20-25 seconds are necessary for mathematical analysis. We prefer to complete three consecutive determinations of cardiac output spaced 1 minute apart. These are averaged; however, in patients receiving mechanical ventilatory support, a similar relationship between the cycling of the mechanical ventilator and the injection of the fluid should be maintained. It is obvious that second-to-second changes in stroke volume do occur and a reproducible technique will eliminate variations in determination of cardiac output which reflect only difference in sampling techniques (18).

There are other sources of potential error. Rapid infusions of cold blood products or even room temperature infusions may affect the baseline and automatic calculation of temperature difference. These should be terminated at least 20 seconds before termination of cardiac output. Vasoactive infusions should not be administered through the injection port utilized for cardiac output determination because the injection would force approximately 1 ml containing the drug into the patient.

Most commercially available instruments contain signals to detect malfunctions such as inadequate battery power, faulty catheter connections, and electronic malfunctions in the thermistor or connecting assemblies. These must be corrected before cardiac output computers can be expected to provide an accurate determination of cardiac output.

Because the computer can only calculate the cardiac output upon the injected sample, it is clear that erroneous calculations may occur if errors are introduced during the procedure. For instance, an inaccurate volume may result in a erroneously high or low cardiac output, dependent upon whether the injection volume is either less than or greater than expected. If the injectate is warmer than sensed by the probe in the control, the computed cardiac output will be higher than is actually present. If the proximal lumen of the pulmonary catheter is not located in the right atrium, the injectate will not be diluted in total cardiac output but will be dispersed in a nonuniform fashion. This may occur in patients of small body habitus so that the distance between the proper positioning of the catheter tip and the right atrium is less than 30 cm. Special catheters may be employed in these situations. Obviously, this is usual in the pediatric age group and special pediatric catheters should be employed. Computation of erroneously low cardiac outputs may occur if a greater volume than expected is introduced and, particularly, if insufficient time lapses between subsequent injections. If the re-equilibration of the entire catheter does not occur, the temperature differential will be overestimated and the numerator will be falsely high, resulting in the overestimation of cardiac output. One-minute delays between injections have been validated as minimal yet sufficient intervals.

Repetitive measurements requiring manipulations of the stopcock seem to impose an additional risk for sepsis. Yet sequential cultures for surveillance have not yet incriminated the technique currently used. Disposable syringes are employed and are used for a single set of three injections. The connecting cable and the thermistor connection are prepared with alcohol and the entire computer and cardiac output cart are cleansed every 24 hours with alcohol. Strict hand washing and clean technique is mandatory.

Other closed systems have been employed using room temperature injectate so that the solution is always connected by a stopcock. A specimen is aspirated through another port of the stopcock and then reinjected. This has apparent advantages in terms of minimizing the measures required to disconnect and directly inject, but we prefer to use iced injectate, and in order to assure consistency and rapid injection, do not inject through a stopcock. Leakage may occur, the rate of injection is often slower and less precisely controlled if the injection is performed through a stopcock. These disadvantages in determining cardiac output are deemed to be of greater importance than the potential of introducing contamination because our system—although frequently studied—has never been implicated as a source of sepsis.

IV. PITFALLS, ERRORS AND REMEDIES

There are a number of unusual situations which may make interpretation of the tracing difficult during insertion and during subsequent use. There are also certain maneuvers that can be used if difficulty is encountered in passing the catheter.

A. Passing a Catheter

Occasionally it is difficult to pass the catheter to the right atrium even if the balloon is immediately inflated upon attaining central venous position. If the conduit has been inserted too far, it is possible that the tip of the conduit actually lies in another central vein and the catheter then will be directed away from the heart. With the balloon inflated and the catheter withdrawn so that the balloon impinges upon the tip of the introducer, the catheter and introducer together can be carefully withdrawn until resistance is felt, indicating that the vessel wall has been reached. The catheter can then be inserted from this position.

In low cardiac output states, the catheter may be difficult to pass because the flow of blood is insufficient to direct the balloon tip. It may be necessary to stimulate cardiac contractions using calcium chloride or beginning an inotropic infusion. If hypovolemia is suspected, a fluid bolus may increase the cardiac output so that the catheter can be passed. Obviously, these are temporizing measures, because the purpose of the catheter itself is to obtain the information to guide further therapy.

I have observed a catheter passed through an atrial septal defect and advanced without the operator's recognition of the situation. The balloon tip was advanced until a "wedge position" was obtained. The catheter was actually lodged in the carotid artery, however, which was obvious from inspection of the postinsertion chest x-ray. It would also be possible for this to occur through a ventricular septal defect. In both these instances, high oxygen tensions would be obtained if specimens were analyzed in the blood gas laboratory.

In cases of right ventricular failure, two abnormalities may occur. Right ventricular end-diastolic pressure may be so high that it might be assumed that this, in fact, represents the pulmonary artery tracing (Figure 2.17). Careful observation of the distance that the catheter is introduced should serve to identify this condition. The catheter tip should be withdrawn to the right atrium and then readvanced. The tracing should be recorded

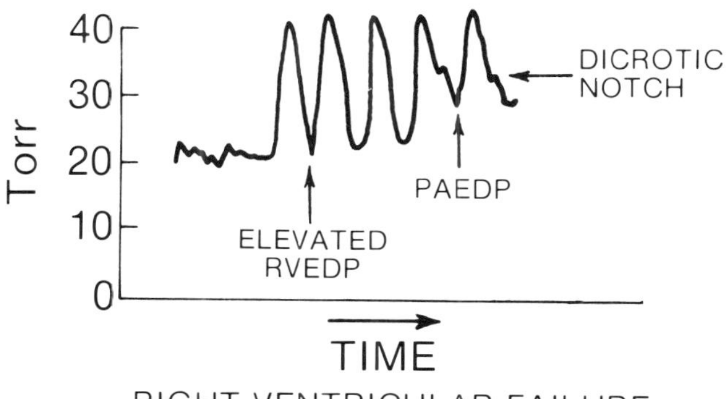

Figure 2.17. Representation of a patient with right ventricular failure. Note that right ventricular end-diastolic pressure exceeds 20 mm Hg. Usually, right ventricular end-diastolic pressure is 10 mm Hg or less. Again, pulmonary artery diastolic pressure itself often is less than 20 mm Hg. It is possible for an inexperienced operator to conclude that this tracing represents pulmonary artery pressures. The absence of the dicrotic notch and the temporal relationship to the right atrial pressure tracing should make this distinction clear.

permanently, if possible, or if the monitor possesses the capability of "freezing the tracing," this should be inspected immediately following introduction into the right ventricle. Additionally, it may be difficult to pass the catheter into the pulmonary artery when either right ventricular failure or marked pulmonary artery hypertension exists. If repeated attempts to traverse the right ventricle are unsuccessful, it may often help to elevate the patient's head 40-50°. In this manner, the balloon may float into the right ventricular outflow tract and ultimately pass into the pulmonary artery.

In patients who suffer hypovolemic shock, extremely low right ventricular and pulmonary artery pressures may be observed. It may be quite difficult to ascertain that, in fact, the catheter has passed into its correct position (Figure 2.18). There will also be an extremely small difference between pulmonary artery diastolic and right ventricular end-diastolic pressure in these conditions. Rapid fluid infusion may make the situation more interpretable, as well as providing primary therapy for the underlying disorder, and should be undertaken as soon as possible. A bubble in the system may cause sufficient damping to produce an identical tracing. The entire system should be inspected to be sure that this tracing is real and not caused by artifact.

B. Interpretation

The most common difficulties, however, occur in situations in which interpretation of the pulmonary artery and wedge tracing is difficult because specific pathophysiologic mechanisms occur. These include any of the following, singly, or in combination: tachycardia, mitral stenosis, mitral insufficiency, chronic obstructive pulmonary disease, and pulmonary hypertension. In patients with severe tachycardia, especially if catheter whip artifact is present, the tracing is extremely "busy." It may be quite difficult to determine an accurate position for measuring wedge pressure (Figure 2.19). In patients with marked pulmonary hypertension, the catheter may be

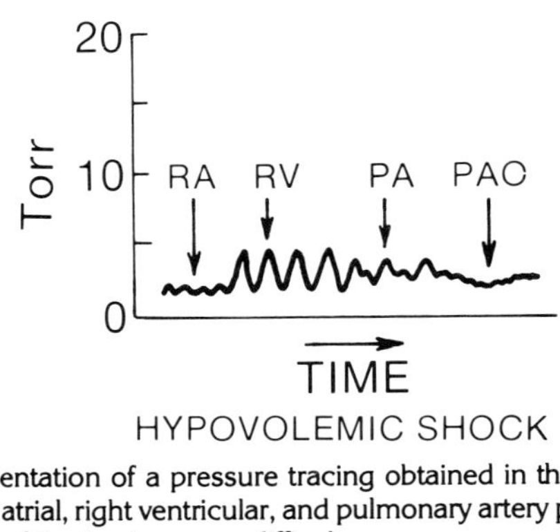

Figure 2.18. Representation of a pressure tracing obtained in the patient in hypovolemic shock. Note that right atrial, right ventricular, and pulmonary artery pressures are all quite low making interpretation of the tracing more difficult.

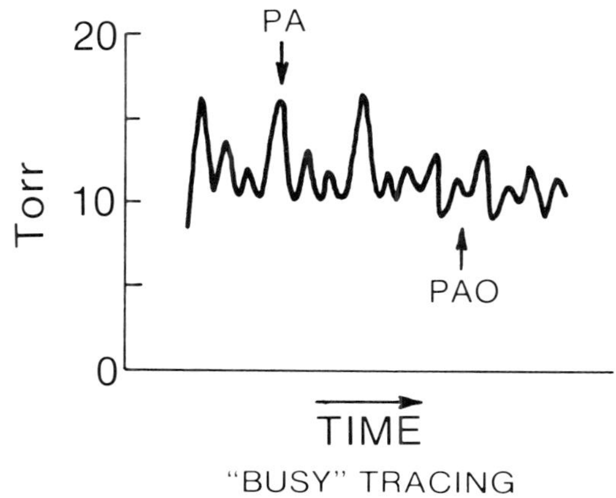

Figure 2.19. A "busy" pulmonary artery tracing. The numerous waveforms make interpretation of the tracing particularly difficult. This can only be resolved by careful inspection of the tracing upon inflation and deflation of the balloon to ascertain that the catheter tip is in an appropriate position to obtain both pulmonary artery and wedge tracings.

difficult to position correctly and, additionally, it is not uncommon that the catheter tip reverses its direction and again traverses the pulmonary valve, leaving a loop in the pulmonary artery. If the catheter is advanced, the tip may impinge upon the right ventricular musculature. The damping of the tracing may be assumed to represent wedge position. Chest x-ray should reveal the course of the catheter. The operator then would be required to reposition the catheter.

In cases of severe mitral insufficiency, the V wave transmitted during systole may, in fact, mimic the pulmonary arterial tracing, making accurate interpretation difficult (Figure 2.20). A continuous electrocardiographic reading should be superimposed on the pressure tracing. When the balloon is inflated and the V wave appears, it should be located later in the cardiac cycle than the pulmonary arterial systolic waveform. Thus, a separation of the waveform can be used to infer the catheter is in correct position. With the balloon inflated, a specimen should be rapidly aspirated for blood gas analysis. If the catheter tip is in correct position, one should obtain a higher oxygen tension representing contamination with capillary blood. In chronic obstructive pulmonary disease with bronchospasm or asthmatic states, the patient may markedly increase intrathoracic pressure during exhalation. This pressure will, of course, be transmitted to the catheter making interpretation of the wedge tracing extremely difficult (Figure 2.21). In one severe case, we noted that the pressure tracing during exhalation exceeded 100 mm Hg. It was not possible to get an accurate wedge pressure reading until the bronchospasm had been treated. Even after treatment, it was clear that this artifact lessened toward the end of exhalation and the wedge

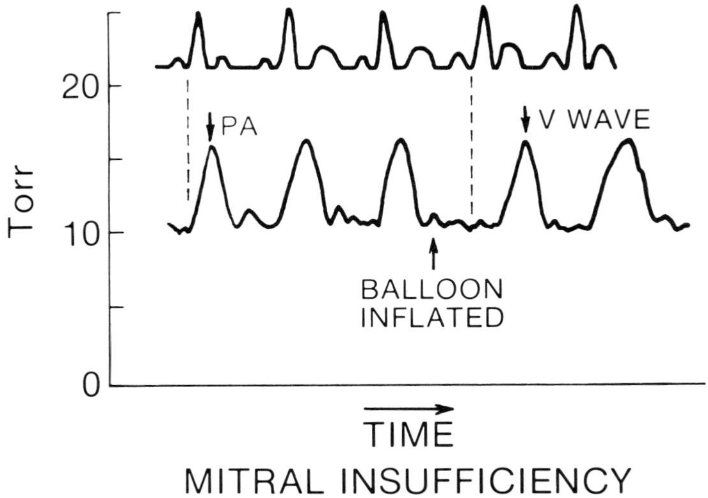

Figure 2.20. Representation of a tracing in a patient with mitral insufficiency. Note the relationship between the QRS complex and the initial deflection of the pulmonary artery tracing. After the balloon has been inflated and the wedge tracing obtained, the V wave "moves away" from the QRS complex.

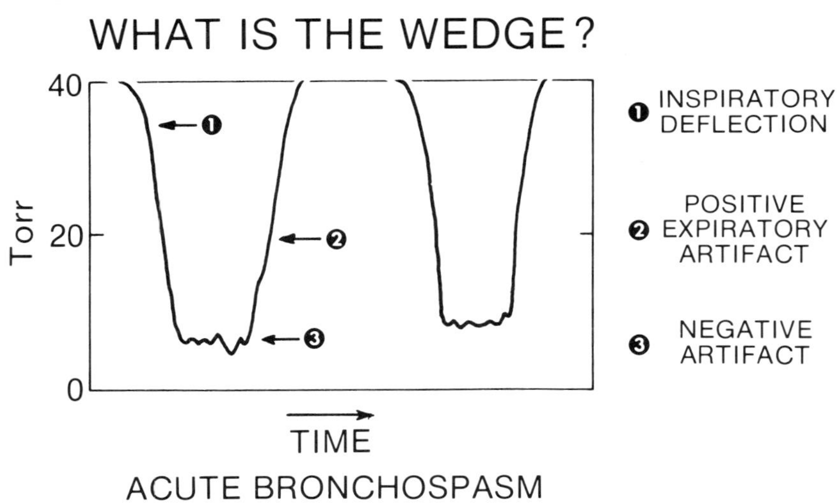

Figure 2.21. A wedge tracing in a patient with severe asthmatic bronchitis and marked elevation of intrathoracic pressure during exhalation due to air trapping. Note that it is impossible to ascertain true wedge pressure at this time. The inspiratory effort resulted in a marked negative deflection of the pressure tracing and the forced exhalation caused a positive pressure artifact that did not permit evaluation of intravascular pressure.

pressure tracing was then interpreted at the last moment of exhalation. At this time, gas flow and pressure changes were minimal as the patient prepared for his next inspiratory effort (Figure 2.22).

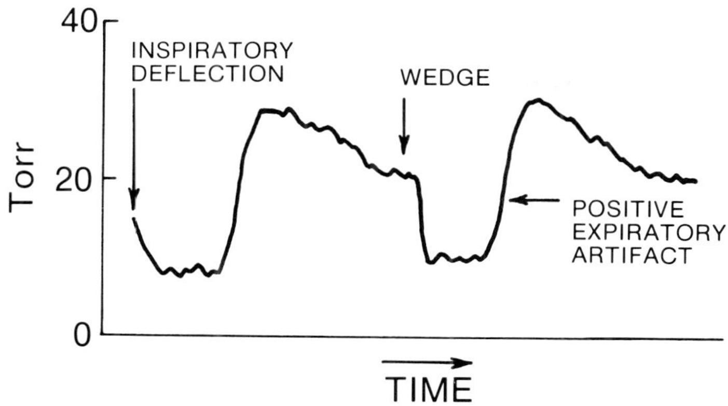

Figure 2.22. Representation of the pressure tracing following treatment of the bronchospasm. Although the negative inspiratory artifact is still visible, the magnitude of the artifact visible during expiration has diminished. At the end of expiration, just before the next inspiratory effort, the pressure consistently returned to the same baseline. Because there was essentially no air flow at this time, this point was chosen to represent true wedge pressure.

Because mitral stenosis usually results in a significant pressure gradient across the mitral valve, interpretation of the wedge pressure in these situations must be made with care, as it no longer represents true left ventricular filling pressure. It may be necessary to empirically determine the optimal wedge pressure by establishing a ventricular function curve and ignore the usual limits of 13-17 torr usually considered to be the optimal range of filling pressure.

Finally, overinflation of the balloon may cause artifactual elevation of the pressure displayed upon the monitor (Figure 2.23).

C. Positioning

It is occasionally desirable to position the catheter in one lung or the other. Usually, catheters pass into a right lower pulmonary artery. However, if one should wish to position the catheter in the left lung, for instance, if a patient is to undergo right pneumonectomy, the likelihood of passing to the left side is enhanced by positioning the patient in the right lateral decubitus position when the catheter is in the right ventricle. The catheter is advanced slowly through the pulmonary valve and slowly advanced to wedge position. In

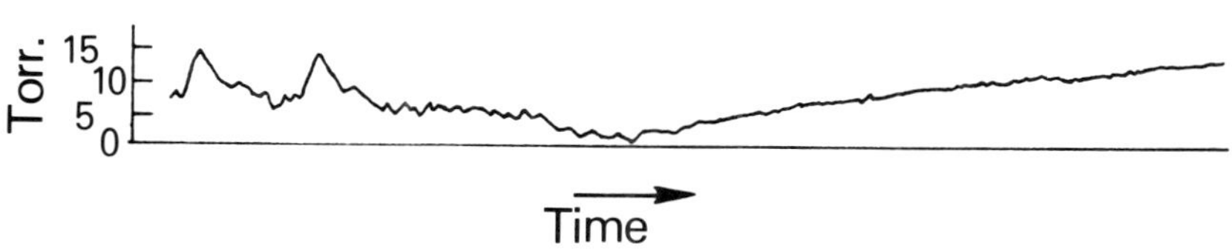

Figure 2.23. If the balloon is overinflated it may either partially occlude the pressure sensing lumen or force the tip of the catheter against the vessel wall—both result in artifactually elevated measurements.

about 80% of the cases, the catheter will enter the left pulmonary artery using this technique. The balloon should be left inflated while the patient's position is changed after insertion and during subsequent positioning on the operating table. In one memorable case these precautions were not observed, even though the catheter had been passed into the appropriate side and confirmed by chest x-ray. During the subsequent operation, the pulmonary artery tracing suddenly disappeared when the surgeon clamped the pulmonary artery. The significance of this change was immediately apparent after the pulmonary artery was amputated and the cut end of the catheter was exposed. Unfortunately, this realization came just after the operator attempted to flush the catheter, which resulted in an unexpected squirt in the face of the surgeon.

V. SUMMARY

Pulmonary artery catheterization has become popular and provides much necessary information. An understanding of the principles of monitoring, including the function of an electronic monitor, assembling an external system, precautions to promote sterility, and an evaluation of the methodology, should diminish the frequency and significance of complications as well as enhance the reliability of the data obtained. It is probably safe to say that incorrect data are worse than none at all because one would be acting upon exact values that were erroneous. It is only by careful attention to many details that most of these pitfalls can be avoided.

REFERENCES

1. Civetta, J. M. 1980. Invasive catheterization. In W. C. Shoemaker, and W. L. Thompsen (eds.). Critical Care—State of the Art, Vol. 1, pp. B1-B47. Society of Critical Care Medicine, Fullerton, Calif.
2. Civetta, J. M. 1971. Clinical utilization of monitoring equipment, NEREM 71-Record, Part 2, pp. 18-25, IEEE Press, Newton, Mass.
3. Swan, H. J., Ganz, W., Forrester, J., Marcus, H., Diamond, G., and Chonette, D. 1970. Catheterization of the heart in man with use of a flow-directed balloon-tipped catheter. N. Engl. J. Med. 283:447-451.
4. Lantiegne, K. C., and Civetta, J. M. 1978. A system for maintaining invasive pressure monitoring. Heart Lung 7:610-621.
5. Applefeld, J. J., Caruthers, T. E., Reno, D. J., and Civetta, J. M. 1978. Assessment of the sterility of long term cardiac catheterization using the thermodilution Swan Ganz catheter. Chest 74:377-380.
6. Blitt, C. 1974. Central venous catheterization via the external jugular vein: a technique employing the "J" wire. JAMA 229:817-818.
7. Civetta, J. M., Gabel, J. C., and Gemer, M. 1972. Internal jugular vein puncture with a margin of safety. Anesthesiology 36:622-623.
8. Wilson, J. N., Grow, J. B., and DeMong, C. V. 1962. Central venous pressure in optimal blood volume maintenance. Arch. Surg. 85:563-578.

9. Civetta, J. M., Gabel, J. C., and Laver, M. B. 1971. Disparate ventricular function in surgical patients. Surg. Forum 22:136-139.
10. Suter, P. M., Lindauer, J. M., Fairley, H. B., and Schlobohm, R. M. 1975. Errors in data derived from pulmonary artery blood gas values. Crit. Care Med. 3:175-181.
11. Caruthers, T. E., Reno, D. J., and Civetta, J. M. 1979. Implications of positive blood cultures associated with Swan Ganz catheters. Crit. Care Med. 7 (Abstract):135.
12. Etling, T. C., and Reno, D. J., 1978. Septicemia rates using Swan Ganz catheters: Influence of duration of catheterization. Crit. Care Med. 6(Abstract):129.
13. Glass, D. D. 1979. Cardiovascular Medications. In: J. M. Civetta (ed.), Intensive Care Therapeutics, Appleton-Century-Crofts, New York.
14. Civetta, J. M. 1977. Cardiopulmonary calculation: A rapid, simple and inexpensive technique. Intens. Care Med. 3(Abstract):206.
15. Civetta, J. M., and Gabel, J. C. 1975. "Pseudocardiogenic" pulmonary edema. J. Trauma 15:143-149.
16. Ganz, W., Donoso, R., Marcus, H. S., Forrester, J. S., and Swan, H. J. C. 1971. A new technique for measurement of cardiac output by thermodilution in man. Am. J. Cardiol. 27:392-396.
17. American Edwards Laboratories, Santa Ana, CA (Cardiac output computer product information).
18. Kirby, R., Perry, J. C., and Calderwood, H. W. 1975. Cardiorespiratory effects of high positive end-expiratory pressure. Anesthesiology 43:533-539.

Chapter 3

Complications of Pulmonary Artery Catheterization

Charles L. Sprung

Bedside hemodynamic monitoring is a recognized procedure performed daily in many hospitals throughout the world. The design of the balloon-tipped flotation catheter serves to minimize the occurrence of complications. The simplicity and low incidence of complications inevitably results in a disregard for the potential risks of this invasive technique. The exact incidence of many of these complications remains unknown. It is quite clear, however, that complications do occur and that they may be fatal.

There are two types of difficulties encountered during pulmonary artery catheterization. The first are complications which may occur despite the fact that an experienced physician is performing the catheterization and the correct technique is used. The second type of complication is usually related to an inexperienced physician inserting a catheter or ignoring the manufacturer's recommendations for catheter placement. Because of the variability in knowledge, background, and skill of the physicians performing these catheterizations, a large number of the second type of complication have occurred. The ensuing discussion focuses on all complications with guidelines to decrease the incidence of the avoidable and unavoidable complications. The major complications of pulmonary artery catheterizations are shown in Table 3.1.

ARRHYTHMIAS

The most common complication of pulmonary artery catheterization is a deviation from the baseline rhythm, including atrial and ventricular arrhythmias and conduction defects (1-22). It is believed that the soft, flexible

Table 3.1. Complications of pulmonary artery catheterization

1.	Arrhythmias
2.	Right bundle branch block
3.	Pulmonary infarction
4.	Pulmonary artery rupture
5.	Cardiac complications
6.	Knotting
7.	Infections
8.	Balloon rupture
9.	CVP placement
10.	Thrombosis
11.	Thrombocytopenia
12.	Miscellaneous

balloon-tipped catheter's design protects patients from the complications of conventional catheters (9). The forces usually concentrated at the tip of the catheter are widely dispersed over the surface of the balloon catheter, thereby minimizing any stimulatory effects. Swan et al. (1) reported an incidence of ventricular arrhythmias of only 13% in their original series of 70 patients. No episodes of sustained ventricular tachycardia occurred. Since that time, authors have reported ventricular arrhythmias during catheterization as rare and unusual (3, 7, 9, 10) or frequent and common (13, 14, 16, 17). The incidence of ventricular ectopy has varied from 1% to 68%, (1, 2, 4, 6, 7, 11, 12, 15-17). Atrial arrhythmias have included atrial fibrillation and atrial flutter with varying block (5), whereas ventricular arrhythmias have included premature ventricular contractions (PVCs) (1, 2, 11-16), sustained ventricular tachycardia (4, 6, 13, 15-17), and ventricular fibrillation (6, 8, 11, 16, 17) with subsequent mortality. Steele and Davies (3) detected no PVCs and no sustained arrhythmias during the catheterization of 103 patients in the cardiac catheterization laboratory. Shaw (12) noted a 37% incidence of multiple unifocal or multifocal PVCs and only one case of ventricular tachycardia in 73 preoperative catheterizations. Elliott et al. (13) demonstrated PVCs in 46% and ventricular tachycardia in 23% of 116 critically ill patients. We have also shown a high incidence of ventricular tachycardia (53%) during pulmonary artery catheterization of the critically ill (17). An example of catheter-induced ventricular tachycardia and ventricular fibrillation is shown in Figure 3.1. Ventricular arrhythmias may occur with displacement of the catheter tip from the main pulmonary artery into the right ventricle and not only during catheterization.

The differences in the reported incidences of ventricular arrhythmias may be attributed to several factors.

1. The larger and stiffer triple-lumen flotation catheter is associated with a higher incidence of PVC than the double-lumen catheter (2).

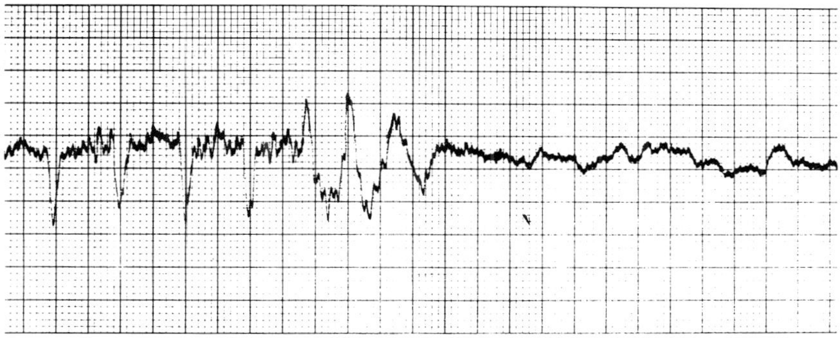

Figure 3.1. Ventricular fibrillation during pulmonary artery catheterization. Note that ventricular fibrillation can occur after a short ventricular salvo and not just after sustained ventricular tachycardia.

2. Several reports have used less than the recommended volume of air (1.5 ml for the 7 French thermodilution catheter) for balloon inflation (12, 13, 15). If the balloon is not properly inflated, it may not completely protrude over the catheter tip during insertion (Figure 3.2). The tip may then traumatize the ventricular endocardial structures.
3. The expertise of the physicians performing the catheterization may affect the frequency of ectopy.
4. The method of recording ventricular ectopy will influence the incidence of arrhythmias. We have shown that merely relying on visual inspection of the electrocardiographic monitor will underestimate the incidence of arrhythmias, including brief episodes of ventricular tachycardia (16). A loud audio signal allows the physician to immediately identify ectopic beats when constant observation of the oscilloscope is impossible.
5. The length of time required for pulmonary artery catheterization may also affect the frequency of arrhythmias. Procedures requiring prolonged catheterization times (patients with severe shock, large right ventricles, tricuspid insufficiency, and pulmonary hypertension) are associated with a higher incidence of ventricular arrhythmias (17). Fluoroscopy may therefore decrease the duration of catheterization and the incidence of arrhythmias by avoiding persistent coiling of the catheter in the right ventricle.
6. Probably most important is the nature of the patient's underlying illness and associated risk factors for the development of ventricular arrhythmias. The previously mentioned studies of patients who were not acutely ill and were undergoing elective catheterization (3, 12) had a lower incidence of ectopy than those of critically ill patients undergoing emergency bedside catheterization (13, 17). In addition, patients with risk factors traditionally known to predispose to ventricular arrhythmias

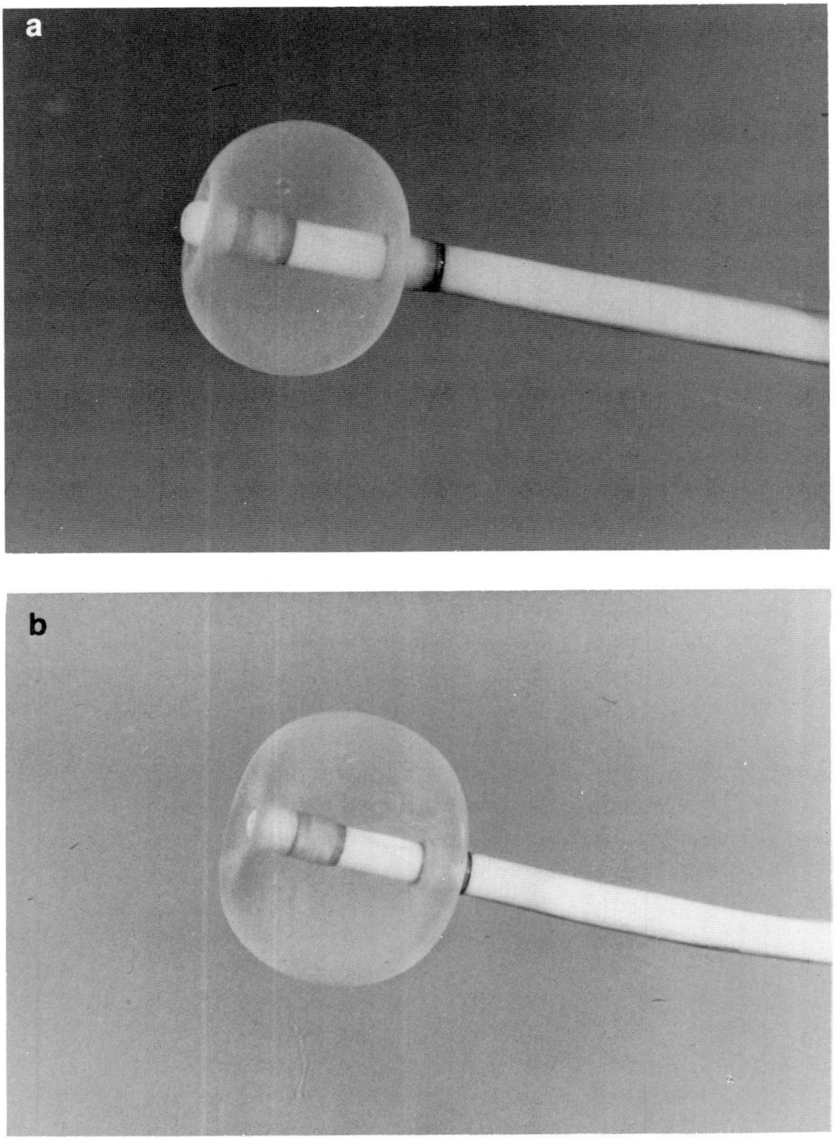

Figure 3.2. Pulmonary artery catheter's (7 French) balloon inflated with 1.0 ml of air (a). The catheter tip remains exposed and trauma to endocardial surfaces may occur during insertion. The same pulmonary artery catheter with the balloon inflated with 1.5 ml of air (b). The balloon protrudes over the catheter tip.

(shock, myocardial ischemia and infarction, hypocalcemia, hypokalemia, hypoxemia, and acidosis) have a significantly higher incidence of ventricular ectopy than those patients without risk factors (17).

Lidocaine has been shown to decrease the incidence of ventricular arrhythmias during passage of the flow-directed balloon-tipped catheter through the right ventricle in patients undergoing elective surgery (12). We have preliminary data demonstrating that prophylactic lidocaine can decrease the incidence of ventricular tachycardia in critically ill patients (18). Therefore, in order to minimize the occurrence of dangerous ventricular arrhythmias during catheterization, the following recommendations are advised:

1. The full 1.5 ml of air should be used for balloon inflation on insertion of 7 French thermodilution catheters (0.8 ml air for 5 French).
2. In addition to visual ECG monitoring, an audio system should be used.
3. Catheterization time should be kept to a minimum; fluoroscopy should be used if available, especially for prolonged catheterizations.
4. If possible, risk factors should be corrected before catheterization, especially acidosis and hypoxemia, which independently correlate with increased ectopy (17).
5. Guidewires and CVP catheters used for insertion of flotation catheters should be cautiously introduced so advancement into the right ventricle does not occur (16).
6. A defibrillator and lidocaine should always be available at the bedside (8). Prophylactic lidocaine may be helpful in decreasing the incidence of ventricular ectopy during catheterization (12, 18).
7. Catheter withdrawal will usually terminate episodes of arrhythmias.
8. All catheters displaced into the right ventricle should be immediately repositioned or removed.
9. High doses of antiarrhythmic medications may be ineffective in treating catheter-induced arrhythmias.

BUNDLE BRANCH BLOCK

The development of a new right bundle branch block has been described during bedside pulmonary artery catheterization with balloon-tipped catheters (13, 17, 19-21). The incidence of catheter-induced right bundle branch block has varied from 3% to 6% and has occurred in patients with and without underlying heart disease (13, 17, 20, 21). The etiology is believed to be either the catheter tip or a rigid catheter loop fixed at the site of venous introduction and at the site of pulmonary artery occlusion, causing mechanical irritation. Therefore, conduction defects as well as arrhythmias may occur during or some time after catheterization. Production of left anterior or posterior fascicular block in addition to right bundle branch block has also been reported (22). These concomitant right- and left-sided conduction defects can be explained by direct trauma to the His bundle (22).

The most serious danger of developing a right bundle branch block is in the patient with pre-existing left bundle branch block who is at risk for the development of complete heart block (19). In fact, Akhtar et al. (23) showed that the incidence of right bundle branch block in the catheterization laboratory is higher in patients with pre-existing left bundle branch block than in patients without this conduction disturbance (23% versus 5%). Our studies have not supported this hypothesis; none of our eight patients with previous left bundle branch block developed a right bundle branch block during bedside catheterization (17).

Some investigators have stressed the need for prophylactic ventricular pacing before pulmonary artery catheterization in patients with baseline left bundle branch block (10, 19). Patients requiring pulmonary artery catheterization, however, are often severely ill and require immediate catheterization. Inserting a pacemaker first would delay the acquisition of important hemodynamic data and might postpone necessary therapeutic interventions. In addition, the placement of a temporary pacemaker would mean a second catheterization and its own inherent risks. Finally, there might be a need for bedside fluoroscopy so that the pulmonary artery catheter would not interfere with the pacemaker wire. Further studies on the incidence and complications associated with pulmonary catheterization in patients with left bundle branch block will be required before recommendations can be made in this group of patients. However, a recent report describes the placement of both catheters through one entry site (24). A 5 French pacemaker catheter is placed into the right ventricle through an 8 French introducer sheath. A guidewire is passed through the same sheath alongside the pacing catheter and the sheath is withdrawn along the pacemaker catheter, freeing the guidewire in the vein. The guidewire is subsequently used for a new introducer and sheath to insert a pulmonary artery catheter. If one decides not to insert a prophylactic pacemaker before pulmonary catheterization of a patient with left bundle branch block, it would be wise to perform the catheterization under fluoroscopy and with a pacemaker present at the bedside.

THROMBOSIS

Thrombus formation may occur with any intravascular catheter. The pulmonary artery flotation catheter is made of polyvinylchloride which does initiate a thrombogenic response. Thrombus formation around or in the pulmonary artery catheter (1, 25-29) and thrombosis of the subclavian, axillary, and jugular venous systems (13, 15, 26, 30, 31) and superior vena cava (27, 32) have been reported. Patients with subclavian venous thrombosis have presented with jugular venous distention and/or upper extremity edema (30). In an early series, thrombosis was the most frequent complication, leading to catheter removal in 23% of cases (25). Recently, Chastre et al. (31) showed venographic or autopsy evidence of internal jugular vein thrombosis at the site of catheter insertion in 22 of 33 patients (66%); no patient had clinical evidence of thrombosis. The demonstration by Hoar et al. of thrombus encapsulating the pulmonary artery catheters of 10 patients undergoing elective catheterization prior to cardiac surgery is also worrisome. All patients developed substantial clots within 60 to 130 minutes of catheter insertion despite heparin pretreatment and flushing of the catheter (28). More recently, Hoar (29) showed that heparin-bonded catheters prevent intraoperative thrombus formation. If thrombosis is so very frequent, one might question the reliability of pressure measurements or thermodilution cardiac output determinations performed with the catheter tip or thermistor covered by thrombus. The clinical importance of these thrombotic episodes and the benefit of heparin-bonded catheters remains uncertain.

Insertion of the pulmonary artery catheter has also been associated with increased platelet consumption and decreased platelet counts (33-35). Foreign surfaces may increase platelet adhesiveness, resulting in clot formation, continued platelet deposition, and subsequent thrombocytopenia. Increased platelet phagocytosis by the reticuloendothelial may also occur. After removal of the catheters, platelet counts begin to increase but remain depressed for 48 hours. Abnormal bleeding has not been associated with catheter-induced thrombocytopenia. Therefore, pulmonary artery catheters should be considered in the differential diagnosis of thrombocytopenia.

PULMONARY DAMAGE

Damage to the pulmonary parenchyma was initially thought to be the most common single group of complications (10), however, 320 recent catheterizations were not associated with evidence of pulmonary infarction or hemorrhage (15). Pulmonary complications are predominantly vascular and include pulmonary infarction (11, 13, 25, 26, 32, 36, 37) and pulmonary artery rupture (38-56).

An early report of pulmonary infarction secondary to flotation catheters showed an incidence of 7.2% (26). Pulmonary infarction may result from (25, 26, 36):

1. Thrombus developing around the catheter and emboli passing through the pulmonary circulation
2. Embolization of thrombus formed within the catheter
3. Occlusion of a branch of the pulmonary artery due to permanent wedging of a distally positioned catheter or prolonged balloon occlusion.

4. Mechanical damage to the pulmonary endothelium by the catheter with subsequent thrombus formation and emboli

The critically ill patient may be particularly prone to this problem. The likelihood of infarction after pulmonary embolism is increased by the presence of pulmonary venous hypertension or systemic hypotension and the lack of bronchial collateral circulation. Therefore, it is not unreasonable to assume that the combination of congestive heart failure, shock, and the mechanical effect of the pulmonary artery catheter in reducing pulmonary blood flow may be sufficient to cause infarction even in the absence of thrombosis (26, 37).

Pulmonary infarction is usually discovered because of clinical signs (hemoptysis and/or other signs of pulmonary emboli) and chest roentgenographic findings (consolidation distal to the catheter tip) (Figure 3.3). Infarction may, however, be totally asymptomatic, and roentgenographic signs of infarction may not develop until several days after the catheter is removed. Involvement of the right lower lobe is most common because the flotation catheter is most often positioned in the intralobar branch of the right pulmonary artery. The extent of the infarction is usually small. Resolution of the x-ray findings usually occurs within 2 to 21 days.

The prevention of pulmonary complications secondary to pulmonary artery catheterization requires meticulous attention to the catheter's insertion and maintenance.

The incidence of pulmonary infarction should be decreased (9, 10, 25, 26,) by:

1. *The use of continuous heparinized flush solution through the pulmonary artery catheter* Scott et al. (25) noted a 23% incidence of thrombosis of catheters prior to the use of a constant heparinized infusion.
2. *Avoidance of persistent wedging of the catheter* Within the first 12 hours of catheter placement, it is common for the catheter to advance further into smaller pulmonary artery branches. This is secondary to the rhythmic contractions of the heart and the pulsatile propelling force of the blood flow. In addition, the catheter softens as it is warmed to body temperature. The loop of catheter around the cardiac structures tends to become smaller and the tip of the catheter moves more peripherally into the pulmonary artery. Foote et al. (26) noted that the catheter tip was situated peripherally in the lung on at least one roentgenogram in 26% of their patients.

   Persistent wedging of the catheter can be avoided by:

   a. Not monitoring the pulmonary artery wedge pressure (PWP) continuously
   b. Measuring the PWP intermittently
   c. Not leaving the catheter in the wedge position for more than 1-2 minutes

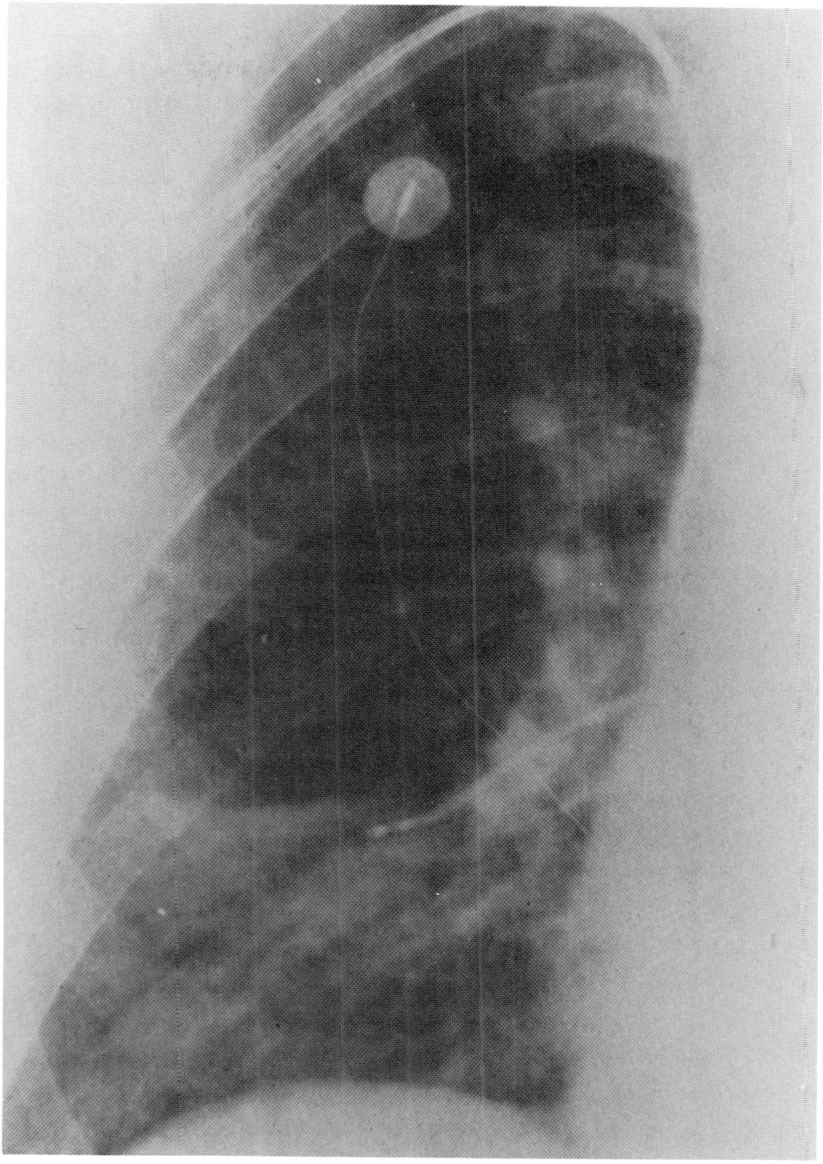

Figure 3.3. Pulmonary infarction from a wedged catheter tip. The area of consolidation extends peripherally from the tip of the catheter. Reproduced from Foote el al., 1974 (26) with permission.

d. Continuously monitoring the pulmonary artery pressure (PA) tracing

e. Making sure a PA tracing is seen when the balloon is deflated (not a PWP or a damped PA tracing)

f. Ascertaining that the volume of air required to inflate the balloon is not substantially less than previously used to obtain a PWP tracing

If a persistent wedge pressure or damped pulmonary artery pressure tracing is found, the catheter should be withdrawn slightly to the proper position.

3. *Determining that the balloon is deflated* Occlusion of a pulmonary artery may occur with the catheter tip in a central portion of a pulmonary artery if the balloon is not deflated after use. This complication may occur despite the air lumen's stopcock being opened to the outside air. If the air lumen is on the inside of a bend in the catheter, the balloon can be inflated normally but air can be trapped beyond the bend (26).
4. *Performing chest roentgenograms immediately after catheter insertion and frequently thereafter to verify the position of the catheter tip and to exclude the possibility of air in the balloon*

PULMONARY ARTERY RUPTURE

In addition to infarction, pulmonary artery rupture should be suspected in any patient with hemoptysis. Cough, dyspnea, or shock may be the presenting symptom, but hemoptysis has been present in 29 of the 32 reported cases (38-41, 43-56).

The incidence of pulmonary artery rupture is 0.2% (55). Roentgenographic changes include infiltrates in the area of the catheter tip or hemothorax. Hemoptysis may range from small amounts of blood-tinged sputum (41, 52) to massive hemorrhage (43, 45, 47, 51).

At least 14 of the 32 reported patients died, five within 30 minutes of symptoms (41, 43, 45, 51, 52). Most of the reported patients have been elderly, with evidence of valvular disease. All but one patient with pressure measurements have had pulmonary hypertension. Twenty of the 32 patients with pulmonary artery rupture have been surgical patients. Fourteen of these patients have had valvular or coronary artery disease. Whether these factors predispose patients to pulmonary artery rupture or whether these factors merely reflect the population of patients requiring catheterization is still unclear. Anticoagulation certainly increases the severity of hemorrhagic complications.

Multiple hypotheses have been proposed for the mechanism of pulmonary artery rupture.

1. A large catheter loop in the right heart predisposes to distal migration of the catheter and possible perforation by the catheter tip (38).
2. Pulmonary artery perforations typically occur at distal bifurcations of the pulmonary artery. Perforation may occur after catheter advancement with an uninflated balloon or by the increased pressure on the pulmo-

nary artery walls caused by balloon inflation in a distal pulmonary branch (41).

3. The pulmonary artery to pulmonary artery wedge pressure gradient produced by balloon inflation might move the catheter more distally in the pulmonary artery, pushing the catheter tip through the vessel wall (39).
4. Pulmonary hypertension distends arterial vessels and causes the catheter to be lodged more peripherally than if pulmonary pressure was normal. Inflation of the balloon in these distended and poorly compliant vessels might cause the tip of the catheter to protrude into the vessel wall. Cardiac pulsations transmitted to the catheter tip might exaggerate any erosions or cause perforation (42).
5. The flotation catheter usually lies in the main pulmonary artery. An inflated balloon catheter advances from the proximal pulmonary artery to the wedge position with great rapidity. This allows a spearing effect to occur with each balloon inflation which could perforate a pulmonary vessel. The stiffer multipurpose catheters might exaggerate these effects (47).
6. The low temperature used during cardiopulmonary bypass in surgical patients may cause the catheter to become extremely rigid. In addition, surgical manipulation of the nondistended heart during bypass may force the deflated catheter tip distally through the pulmonary artery wall. Because the lungs are excluded from the circulation during cardiopulmonary bypass, the perforation may remain unrecognized until the reinstitution of pulmonary blood flow after bypass. Therefore, one must consider the complication of pulmonary artery rupture before routinely performing pulmonary artery catheterization in surgical patients.

Because the catheter tip does not normally protrude beyond the fully inflated balloon, it has been thought that hypotheses 3-5 could be invoked only if the balloon was partially inflated. Unfortunately, this is not necessarily true. Eccentric balloon inflation typically occurs in peripherally located catheters and can cause the catheter tip to impinge on the pulmonary vessel wall (44, 56). The protective effect of the balloon may be lost when the balloon becomes wedged in a tube or pulmonary artery, as demonstrated in Figure 3.4 (42, 47, 56).

Unfortunately, the differentiation between pulmonary infarction and pulmonary artery rupture may not be simple (57-59). Both present with hemoptysis and chest roentgenographic findings. Even in those patients with suspected pulmonary artery rupture, it may not be possible to identify the actual arterial laceration on pathologic examination (43, 45). Most patients with pulmonary infarction have minimal hemoptysis and chest roentgenographic evidence of a localized, nonprogressive pulmonary infiltrate.

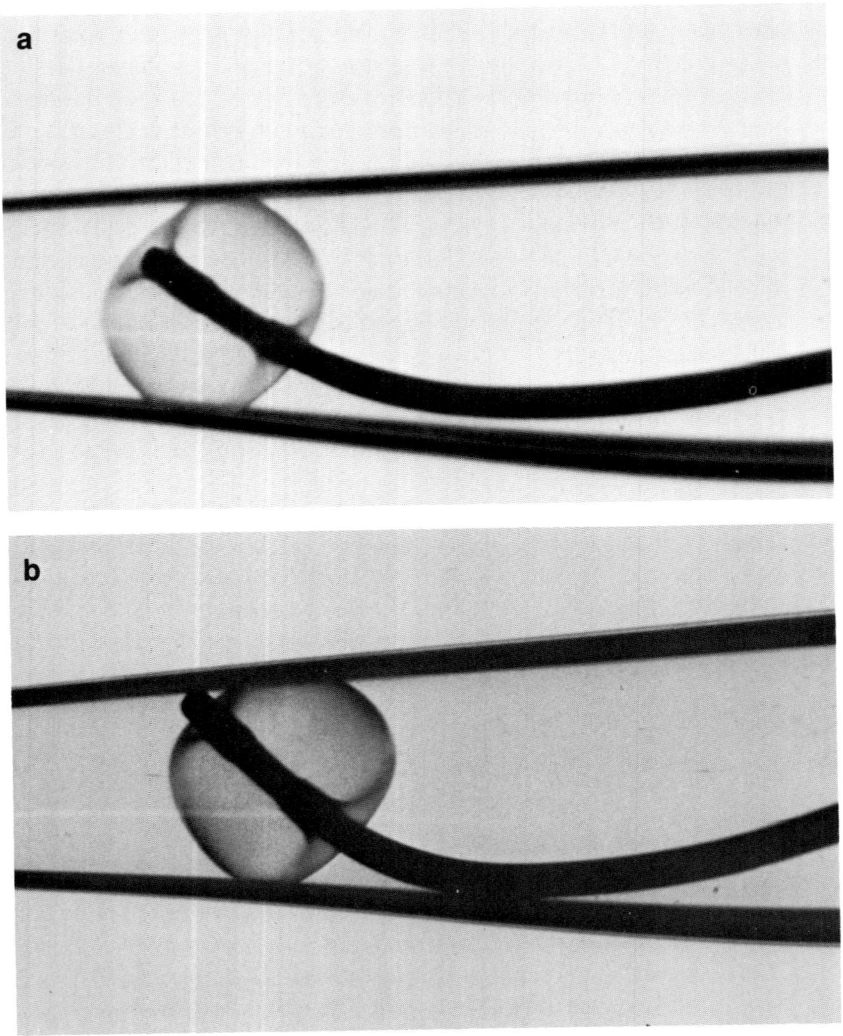

Figure 3.4. Fully inflated balloon tipped catheter (1.5 ml) meeting the lumen of a glass tube (a). The same fully inflated balloon tipped catheter (1.5 ml) with continued insertion (b). The catheter tip protrudes beyond the fully inflated balloon into the "vessel" wall.

Hemothorax is more indicative of pulmonary artery rupture than pulmonary infarction. Aspiration of air through the distal lumen of the catheter is indicative of pulmonary artery rupture (40). The treatment of catheter-induced pulmonary infarction can usually be conservative. Removal or repositioning of the pulmonary catheter and close observation of the vital signs and chest roentgenogram usually suffice.

Patients with pulmonary artery rupture, however, may present with severe hemorrhage. These patients usually require more aggressive management as many of the deaths occur within 30 minutes. The severity of bleeding and the patient's status will dictate the steps to be taken. The patient's affected side (usually the right) should be placed down to prevent the spilling of blood into the unaffected side. Adequate ventilation must be assured with a double-lumen endotracheal tube or intubation of the uninvolved lung when severe hemorrhage occurs. An immediate chest x-ray will grossly localize the bleeding site. Injection of radiographic contrast media through the catheter may further localize the site of bleeding and confirm the diagnosis (46). The catheter should be withdrawn from the site of injury to prevent further bleeding caused by additional pulmonary artery damage by the catheter. Flexible bronchoscopy may identify the bleeding site and permit tamponade. Injection of clotted blood through the pulmonary artery catheter may also be therapeutic (46). However, time may only permit emergency thoracotomy with resection of the involved segment or lobe (58).

Swan and Ganz have emphasized the importance of understanding and observing the manufacturer's detailed instructions for the prevention of complications (60, 61). Nevertheless, the majority of the reports of pulmonary artery rupture have occurred when these guidelines were not followed. Therefore, the following recommendations for the prevention of pulmonary artery rupture should be adhered to (39, 41, 42, 45, 52):

1. Inflate the balloon in a large caliber vein and float the catheter into the pulmonary artery and wedge position. After deflating the balloon, slowly reinflate the balloon until the pulmonary artery pressure tracing changes to a wedge tracing. If the full inflation volume necessary to obtain a wedge pressure is significantly less than recommended (0.5 ml for 4 French, 0.8 ml for 5 French, and 1.5 ml for 7 French), gradually pull back the catheter to a position in which full or near full inflation volume is required to record a pulmonary artery wedge pressure tracing (1.0-1.5 ml for 7 French). If the full inflation volume is required to record a wedge pressure tracing, slightly advance the catheter and check the catheter position again by slowly inflating the balloon. Do not advance the catheter uninflated and later inflate it.
2. Always inflate the balloon for a wedge pressure recording slowly and under continuous pulmonary artery pressure monitoring. Stop inflation immediately upon the pulmonary artery pressure tracing changing to a wedge pressure tracing.
3. Do not inflate the balloon with fluid.
4. Keep the wedge time to a minimum, (2-3 respiratory cycles or 10-15 seconds) especially in patients with pulmonary hypertension.
5. The catheter should be kept in the most central portion of the pulmonary artery, allowing the catheter to float into the wedged position with each balloon inflation.

6. Keep a syringe on the balloon lumen of the catheter to prevent accidental injection of fluids.
7. Avoid excessive catheter manipulation.
8. Reposition or remove the catheter if hemoptysis occurs. Even small amounts may signify rupture or infarction.

Other pulmonary complications include catheter placement in the pleural space (62) and hydromediastinum secondary to fluid infusion through a proximal lumen located outside the venous system (63). This latter complication occurred in a patient of small body habitus using the central approach to the internal jugular vein.

CARDIAC COMPLICATIONS

Lesions of the right atrial endocardium, tricuspid valve, chordae tendineae, and pulmonic valve with subsequent valvular insufficiency have been reported in patients after pulmonary artery catheterization (13, 64-70). Hemorrhage into one or more valve cusps or the actual separation of valvular tissue may occur. Endocardial lesions have had linear configurations consistent with involvement along the course of the catheter. Withdrawal of the catheter with the balloon inflated or forced withdrawal against constant resistance has damaged the chordae tendineae, papillary muscles, or tricuspid valve (67, 70). Septic endocarditis and aseptic thrombotic endocarditis have also been reported (13, 64-66, 68). The incidence has varied from 3.4% to 21% (13, 65, 66). Two series have shown a higher incidence of right sided aseptic thrombotic endocarditis in patients with pulmonary artery catheters when compared to patients not requiring catheterization (65, 66). A recent report demonstrated evidence of endocarditis in six consecutive burn patients who expired (68). Whether the burn patient with a hyperdynamic hemodynamic state and hypercoagulability is at increased risk for endocarditis remains unknown. The constant pumping of the heart against an indwelling catheter may traumatize the endocardium and cause mural thrombi. Endocarditis may increase the risk for subsequent embolization or infection. It is believed that prolonged catheterization may contribute to cardiac complications. Patients with these complications have had their catheters in place for prolonged periods of time, usually longer than 3 days (66, 68, 69).

The prevention of these complications entails:

1. Catheter withdrawal with the balloon deflated
2. Never forcing the withdrawal of the catheter when resistance is encountered
3. Avoiding prolonged catheterization

KNOTTING

Knotting of a pulmonary artery catheter can occur within the vascular space (71-75) or around cardiac structures (70, 76-80). The flotation catheter can also be caught in suture material placed through the right atrial wall during cardiac surgery (79, 81, 82). Knotting is more common with small-bore flotation catheters. Kinking and looping, which are the precursors of knotting, occur when an excessive length of catheter is inserted. After a right ventricular pressure tracing has appeared during insertion, not more than 10-15 cm of catheter should be required to obtain a pulmonary artery pressure tracing. Dilated heart chambers and repeated catheter manipulation especially without fluoroscopy are predisposing factors. Catheter insertion without balloon inflation will not only predispose to coiling in the right ventricle, but may cause lodging of the catheter between the right ventricular wall and the chordae tendineae. Figure 3.5 is an example of catheter looping and knotting.

The possibility of knot formation must be considered whenever resistance is encountered on withdrawal of an intravascular catheter. When tension is applied to the catheter attached to a cardiac structure, tugging may be felt with each contraction (77). Chest x-ray or fluoroscopy will reveal the site of the loop or knot. Other clues include a "damped" pulmonary artery pressure tracing or the inability to obtain a satisfactory pulmonary artery wedge pressure tracing despite repeated flushing. Ventricular arrhythmias occurring simultaneously with right atrial pressure recordings may indicate that the catheter tip is in the right atrium and a loop is present in the right ventricle.

To prevent looping and knotting, the following guidelines should be followed:

1. Fully inflate the balloon in a large central vein before advancing the catheter to the right atrium.
2. Do not use excessive length of the pulmonary artery catheter for insertion. If the pulmonary artery pressure tracing is not obtained after 15 cm of catheter has been introduced into the right ventricle, withdraw the catheter to the right atrium, do not advance further.
3. If possible, use fluoroscopy especially in patients with dilated cardiac chambers.
4. Remove the first pulmonary artery catheter after a second is introduced into a central vein.

In general, catheters are difficult to unknot if they are not loose and if they are located a distance from the catheter tip. The removal of a catheter should never be forced when resistance is encountered. Continued resistance may indicate catheter attachment to an intracardiac structure. Forced

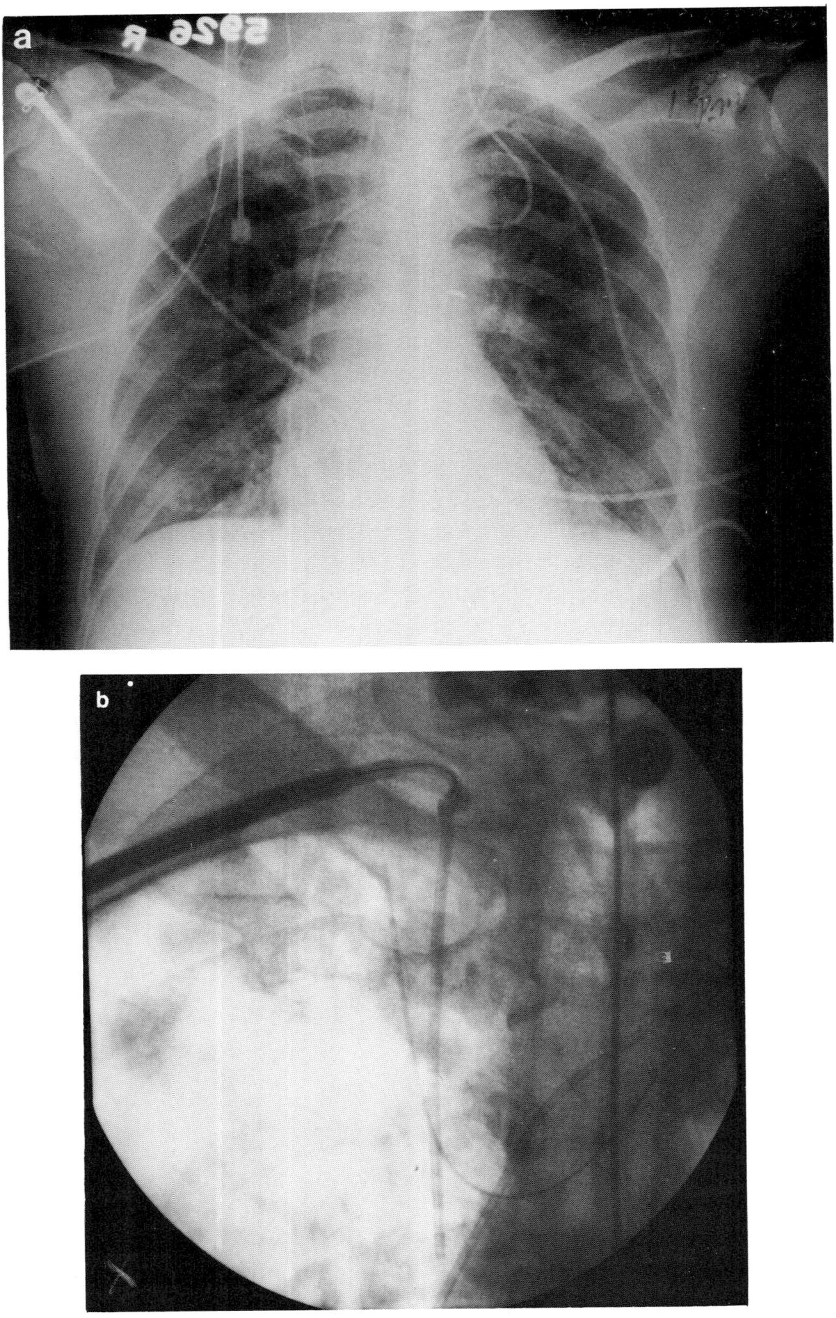

Figure 3.5. Catheter looping in the right ventricle (a). Pulmonary artery catheter knotting and removal (b). Reproduced from Dach et al., 1981 (75) with permission.

removal may cause avulsion of the tricuspid valve, papillary muscle, or chordae tendineae (70). If knotting does occur, one can use one of several techniques to remove the catheter. The less invasive methods are usually attempted initially.

1. Gentle traction may allow withdrawal of the catheter directly from the vein or through a more proximal cutdown (71, 76).
2. Under fluoroscopy, the catheter can be manipulated into numerous positions in order to loosen and move the knot toward and over the catheter tip (74).
3. If the knot is not tight, a movable cord guidewire can be directed along the major lumen of the catheter. The adjustable inner core of the guidewire can be used to stiffen the distal part and the knot can be loosened or made to spring open. Passage of a semiflexible guidewire through the catheter lumen is ineffective in complete knotting and may be hazardous as perforation of the catheter, blood vessel, or heart could occur (74).
4. Picking at the knot with a firm catheter may also be useful (76).
5. A knot or suture can be tightened against a relatively rigid venous sheath or Teflon sleeve introduced over the external portion of the catheter permitting its easy withdrawal (80, 81). In addition, the distal end of the catheter can be manipulated with a pigtail catheter or stone retriever basket into the inferior vena cava and brought to the outside. The application of forceful pulling from both ends of the catheter can tighten the knot which can be withdrawn through a saphenous vein (79).
6. Dilating the puncture site with 10 and 14 French dilators from a biliary stent kit and pulling the knot tightly against the end of the catheter has recently been reported (75) (Figure 3.5b).
7. If the knot is wrapped around a cardiac structure, thoracotomy and cardiotomy may be required for its removal (74, 79).
8. In the nonsurgical candidate, permanent catheter retention is a possible alternative (76, 78). The catheter has been sutured to the vein and surrounding fascia in a patient and left in place for 16 months without sequela (76). The various retrieval devices are shown in Figure 3. 6.

INFECTIOUS COMPLICATIONS

Patients with pulmonary artery catheters are particularly vulnerable to bacterial contamination and severe infection because of the catheters' intracardiac location and repeated break of a closed infusion system. In addition to constant pressure measurements, blood is aspirated for central venous and mixed venous blood samples and cold solutions are injected for thermodilution cardiac output determinations. Many series have sought to determine

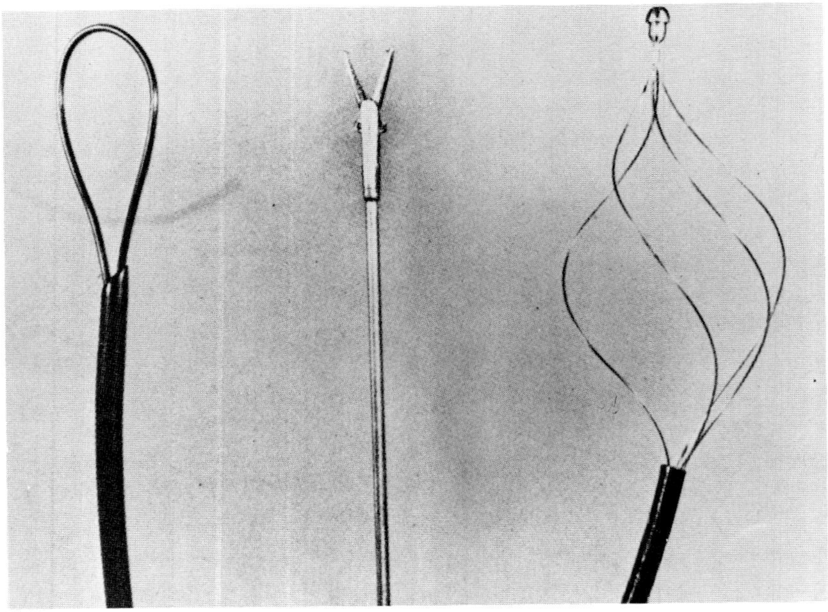

Figure 3.6. Devices for retrieval of intracardiac foreign bodies. *Left*, an adjustable loop snare. *Center*, bronchoscopic grasping forceps. *Right*, modified urologic basket stone catcher. Reproduced from Dotter et al., 1971. Transluminal extraction of catheter and guidewire fragments from the heart and great vessels: 29 collected cases. Am. J. Roentgenol. 111:467, with permission.

the incidence of infectious complications of pulmonary artery catheterization (11, 13-15, 65, 68, 83, 84). Unfortunately, it is often difficult to differentiate between contamination, colonization, and actual infection. Elliott et al. (13) provide guidelines for defining infectious problems related to pulmonary artery catheters.

1. *Colonization* is defined by a positive culture of the catheter without evidence of local or systemic infection.
2. *Colonization with potential infection* is defined by a positive culture of the catheter with clinical manifestations of local tissue invasion or sepsis.
3. *Contamination* is defined as one of multiple blood cultures yielding a typical nonpathogen and culture of the catheter failing to grow the same organism.

In cases of infection, the role of the pulmonary artery catheter can be designated as:

1. *Definite*—positive blood cultures and histologic or bacteriologic proof of the same bacteria at the catheter site with no other site of infection.

2. *Probable*—same organism recovered from the catheter and from the blood stream with another possible focus.
3. *Unrelated*—same organism recovered previously from another site thought to be the primary source of infection.

Applefeld et al. (83) observed a colonization rate of 9% in elective surgical patients requiring catheterization as compared to 46% for patients with identifiable sources of sepsis prior to catheterization. All peripheral blood cultures in the 57 patients were negative. Patients with colonization had an increased duration of catheterization, a greater number of catheter repositioning, and a greater number of catheterizations per patient. Colonization increased after 72 hours of catheter use and after three repositions. The same investigators noted a 3% incidence of catheter-related infection in a larger group of patients (84). Elliott et al. (13) noted a 35% incidence of colonization. The pulmonary artery catheter was the probable source of septicemia in 2% of the 116 catheterizations. Prolonged catheterization did not increase the incidence of positive catheter cultures. Puri et al. (14) noticed a 3% colonization rate in their 71 patients. Sise et al. (15) noted septic sequela (defined as positive blood cultures thought to have originated from the catheter site or by a spiking temperature curve which subsided after catheter removal) in 8% of 320 catheterizations. Infections at the catheter site and septic sequela were rare before 72 hours and increased significantly after that time. Preexisting central venous sites were used for insertion in 67% of patients. Interestingly, there was no difference in the incidence of cellulitis or infection between catheters in new or preexisting central venous sites. Finally, several reports have noted bacterial endocarditis of the tricuspid or pulmonary valves and septic emboli (65, 68). In addition, one patient had a myocardial abscess (68).

Repositioning the pulmonary artery catheter by withdrawal from the wedge position should not increase infectious complications. However, advancing a catheter forward represents a deviation from standard surgical technique and could increase infectious problems. Some physicians have recommended replacing the catheter through the original venous site if advancement is necessary (85). Most physicians, however, advance catheters after some type of "sterilization" and do not replace them. As central venous catheters may become colonized in the fibrin sleeve along their intravenous course, utilization of the original insertion site for catheter replacement might increase the risk of infection. If replacement is deemed necessary, a new venipuncture site and catheterization is required (86). The use of a plastic sheath around the catheter and introducer may maintain sterility despite catheter manipulation (87). These sheaths are now commercially available.

Prevention of infectious complications is important. Strict sterile technique should be used routinely for catheterization. Masks and gowns are worn during catheterization. Topical antibiotic ointment is applied at the insertion site and sterile dressings are used. For long-term monitoring, percutaneous catheter insertion is recommended as more infections occur at cut-down sites. The catheter should be removed as soon as possible. If the catheter is believed to be a source of infection, it should also be removed. Infectious complications increase after 72 hours of catheterization and multiple repositioning. The morbidity and mortality of prolonged catheterization or a repositioned catheter must be weighed against the hazards of a new insertion and catheterization.

BALLOON RUPTURE

Balloon rupture has been reported in 1% to 23% of pulmonary artery catheterizations (1, 6, 12, 13, 15, 88, 89). It is important to test the catheter and balloon before catheterization because as many as 3% of catheters will have ruptured balloons or incompetent channels prior to catheterization (15). We have experienced a lower incidence. Balloon incompetence may vary from tiny perforations to frank rupture. The balloon is made of latex which absorbs lipoproteins from the blood, leading to a loss of the balloon's elasticity. Balloon rupture has been associated with catheters undergoing repeated uses, exceeding the recommended balloon inflation volumes, catheterization for prolonged times, multiple inflations, and withdrawal of the catheter through the introducer with an inflated balloon (1, 6, 12, 89). Shaw has suggested that two holes can be bored into the barrel of a 2- or 3-ml syringe at the 1.5-ml mark of the syringe for use with 7 French flotation catheters. This would prevent overinflation of the balloon because any attempt to use more than 1.5 ml of air would result in the loss of the excess volume through the side ports (12). Inflation is usually associated with a feeling of resistance. On release, the plunger of the syringe typically springs back and the balloon deflates. It is not usually necessary to actively deflate the balloon. In fact, active deflation may decrease the life span of the balloon. If no resistance to inflation is encountered, it should be assumed that the balloon has ruptured. Thereafter, inflation should no longer be performed. Under normal circumstances, air is used as the inflation medium for the balloon. The use of air has not caused any major problem; it appears that 0.8-1.5 cc of air does not produce adverse effects if injected into the pulmonary artery. Carbon dioxide, which is much more soluble in blood, should be used as the inflation medium in patients who might have a right-to-left shunt. Another potential complication of balloon rupture is fragmentation of the balloon and subsequent embolization. Patients with balloon rupture of their catheters may require recatheterization, particularly if the pulmonary artery diastolic pressures do not correlate with the pulmonary artery wedge pressure.

The following recommendations should help avoid balloon rupture and the need for repeat catheterization.

1. Test the integrity of the balloon and catheter before catheterization.
2. Use catheters only once.
3. Do not exceed recommended inflation volumes. Placing holes in a syringe at the 1.5-ml mark may be helpful in 7 French catheters.
4. Passively deflate the balloon by removing the inflating syringe.
5. Avoid multiple balloon inflations unless necessary. The balloon is usually inflated hourly to obtain a pulmonary artery wedge pressure but may be inflated every 15-30 seconds if required.
6. Do not continue inflation against a persistent resistance.
7. Remove catheters as soon as possible.
8. Do not withdraw a catheter through an introducer with the balloon inflated.
9. As soon as the catheter is placed, correlate the pulmonary artery diastolic pressure with the pulmonary artery wedge pressure.

CVP PLACEMENT

Complications of pulmonary artery catheterization include those complications of any central venous catheter placement. These include bleeding (12, 14, 15), hematoma, pain and swelling, inflammation (15), infection (14, 15, 83, 84, 88), thrombophlebitis (4), arterial puncture (11, 15), pneumothorax (11), hemothorax or hydrothorax (11), air embolism (90), thoracic duct injury, and brachial nerve injury (11).

MISCELLANEOUS

Other complications of pulmonary artery catheterization include the Bernard-Horner syndrome (91), placement of the catheter tip into the wall of the internal carotid artery (92), massive hematuria (93), pneumoperitoneum (94), fracture of a flotation catheter with an inability to obtain an acceptable wave form (95), and separation of the hub and shaft of an introducer with the shaft disappearing into the venous system (62). Guidewires may be lost into the venous system.

Table 3.2 lists the known complications of pulmonary artery catheterization, the factors predisposing to their development and the possible precautions to prevent their occurrence.

Considering the frequent use of the pulmonary artery catheter, the reported morbidity and mortality remains remarkably low. However, many

Table 3.2. Predisposing factors and precautions in the prevention of complications

Complication	Cause and/or predisposing factor	Prevention and/or precaution
1. Arrhythmia	1. Irritation of endocardium or heart valves by catheter	Monitor ECG continuously during insertion
	2. Looping or knotting of excess catheter in RV	Avoid over-manipulation
	3. Catheter falling back into RV from PA	Keep lidocaine and defibrillator on hand
	4. Inadequate balloon inflation during insertion	Fully inflate balloon (1.5 ml for 7F)
	5. Prolonged catheterization	? Fluoroscopy
	6. Underlying disease	
	7. Risk factors	Correct acidosis, hypoxemia, electrolyte abnormality
		Catheter withdrawal if arrhythmias are noted
		? Prophylactic lidocaine
2. Complete heart block	1. Previous left bundle branch block	? Prophylactic pacemaker Fluoroscopy
3. Thrombosis		Continuous flush with heparinized solution
		? Heparin-bonded catheters
4. Pulmonary Infarction	1. Persistent wedging of a distally portioned catheter	Avoid persistent wedging Measure PA continuously Monitor PWP intermittently for short periods
		Air requirement for balloon inflation should remain constant
		Catheter withdrawal if persistent wedge or damped PA
	2. Prolonged balloon occlusion	Maintain balloon deflated
		Frequent chest x-rays
		Never flush catheter if clotting suspected
5. Pulmonary Artery Rupture	1. Catheter advancement with uninflated balloon	Do not advance catheter uninflated and later inflate.
	2. Balloon inflation in distal pulmonary artery	Slowly inflate to a PWP under continuous PA monitoring

Table 3.2. (continued)

Complication	Cause and/or predisposing factor	Prevention and/or precaution
		Stop inflation immediately when PWP obtained Keep PWP time to a minimum (10-15 sec) Avoid excess catheter manipulation Avoid flushing catheter forcefully in wedge position Keep catheter in a central portion of the PA If permanent PWP, pull back to PA
	3. Balloon inflation with fluid	Do not inflate balloon with fluid
	4. Large catheter loop in the right heart	Do not use excessive catheter length
	5. Pulmonary hypertension	
	6. Elderly	
	7. Valvular disease	
6. Cardiac	1. Catheter withdrawal with the balloon inflated	Withdraw catheter with balloon deflated
	2. Forced withdrawal against resistance	Do not force withdrawal
	3. Prolonged catheterization	Remove catheter as soon as possible
7. Knotting	1. Small bore catheters	
	2. Excessive catheter length	Do not use excessive catheter length for insertion Insert a maximum of 15 cm of catheter from the RV to PA
	3. Insertion with deflated balloon	Fully inflate balloon before insertion
	4. Repeated manipulation in dilated heart	? Fluoroscopy
8. Infections	1. Increased duration of catheterization (> 72 hours)	Remove catheter as soon as possible
	2. Increased catheter repositioning	Avoid repositioning if possible
	3. Increased catheterizations	? Plastic sheath Percutaneous insertion

Table 3.2. (continued)

Complication	Cause and/or predisposing factor	Prevention and/or precaution
		Insert new catheter at new site
	4. Inadequate sterilization	Strict sterile technique
		Frequent change of dressing and IV connections
9. Balloon Rupture	1. Repeated catheter use	Test balloon before insertion
		Use catheter once
	2. Balloon inflation volumes exceeding recommendations	Do not exceed recommended inflation volumes
		Do not inflate against persistent resistance
	3. Prolonged catheterization	Remove catheter as soon as possible
	4. Multiple balloon inflations	Inflate balloon only when required
	5. Catheter withdrawal through the introducer with the balloon inflated	Do not withdraw catheter with the balloon inflated
		If balloon is ruptured, it should not be filled with air

complications are probably not reported. The true incidence of complications of pulmonary artery catheterization will remain unknown until a large prospective multicenter study is performed. Despite the benefits of the pulmonary artery catheter, complications and even mortality are real concerns. Each catheterization must be evaluated individually and the risks must be weighed against the potential benefits.

REFERENCES

1. Swan, H. J. C., Ganz, W., Forrester, J., Marcus, H., Diamond, G., and Chonette, D. 1970. Catheterization of the heart in man with use of a flow-directed balloon-tipped catheter. N. Engl. J. Med. 283:447-451.
2. Forrester, J. S., Diamond, G. A., and Swan, H. J. C. 1972. Bedside diagnosis of latent cardiac complications in acutely ill patients. JAMA 222:59-63.
3. Steele, P., and Davies, H. 1973. The Swan-Ganz catheter in the cardiac laboratory. Brit. Heart J. 35:647-650.
4. Mond, H. G., Hunt, D., and Sloman, G. 1973. Hemodynamic monitoring in the coronary care unit using the Swan-Ganz right heart catheter. Brit. Heart J. 35:635-642.
5. Geha, D. G., Davis, N. J., and Lappas, D. G. 1973. Persistent atrial arrhythmias

associated with placement of a Swan-Ganz catheter. Anesthesiology 39:651-653.
6. Archer, G., and Cobb, L. A. 1974. Long term pulmonary artery pressure monitoring in the management of the critically ill. Ann. Surg. 180:747-752.
7. Voukydis, P. C., and Cohen, S. I. 1974. Catheter-induced arrhythmias. Am. Heart J. 88:588-592.
8. Cairns, J. A., and Holder, D. 1975. Ventricular fibrillation due to passage of a Swan-Ganz catheter. Am. J. Cardiol. 35:589.
9. Swan, H. J. C., and Ganz, W. 1975. Use of balloon flotation catheters in critically ill patients. Surg. Clin. North Am. 55:501-520.
10. Swan, H. J. C. 1975. The role of hemodynamic monitoring in the management of the critically ill. Crit. Care Med. 3:83-89.
11. Katz, J. D., Cronau, L. H., Barash, P. G., and Mandel, S. D. 1977. Pulmonary artery flow-guided catheters in the perioperative period: Indications and complications. JAMA 237:2832-2834.
12. Shaw, T. J. I. 1979. The Swan-Ganz pulmonary artery catheter. Anaesthesia 34:651-656.
13. Elliott, C. G., Zimmerman, G. A., and Clemmer, T. P. 1979. Complications of pulmonary catheterization in the care of critically ill patients. Chest 76:647-652.
14. Puri, V. K., Carlson, R. W., Bander, J. J., and Weil, M. H. 1980. Complications of vascular catheterization in the critically ill: A prospective study. Crit. Care Med. 8:495-499.
15. Sise, M. J., Hollingsworth, P., Brimm, J. E., Peters, R. M., Virgilio, R. W., and Shackford, S. R. 1981. Complications of the flow-directed pulmonary-artery catheter: A prospective analysis in 219 patients. Crit. Care Med. 9:315-318.
16. Sprung, C. L., Jacobs, L. J., Caralis, P. V., and Karpf, M. 1981. Ventricular arrhythmias during Swan-Ganz catheterization of the critically ill. Chest 79:413-415.
17. Sprung, C. L., Pozen, R. G., Rozanski, J. J., Pinero, J., Eisler, B. R., and Castellanos, A. 1982. Advanced ventricular arrhythmias during bedside pulmonary artery catheterization. Am. J. Med. 72:203-208.
18. Sprung, C. L., Garcia, A. A., Sequeira, R. F., and Marcial, E. H. 1982. The use of prophylactic lidocaine to prevent ventricular tachycardia during pulmonary artery catheterization—A double blind, prospective, randomized study. Crit. Care Med. 10(Abstract):218.
19. Abernathy, W. S. 1974. Complete heart block caused by the Swan-Ganz catheter. Chest 65:349.
20. Luck, J. C., and Engel, T. R., 1976. Transient right bundle branch block with "Swan-Ganz" catheterization. Am. Heart J. 92:263-264.
21. Thomson, I. R., Dalton, B. C., Lappas, D. G., and Lowenstein, E. 1979. Right bundle-branch block and complete heart block caused by the Swan-Ganz catheter. Anaesthesiology 51:359-362.
22. Castellanos, A., Ramirez, A. V., Mayorga-Cortes, A., Pefkaros, K., Rozanski, J. J., Sprung, C. L., and Myerburg, R. J. 1981. Left fascicular blocks during right-heart catheterization using the Swan-Ganz catheter. Circulation 64:1271-1276.
23. Akhtar, M., Damato, R. N., Gilbert-Leeds., C. J., Batsford, W. P., and Reddy, C. P. 1977. Induction of iatrogenic electrocardiographic patterns during electrophysiologic studies. Circulation 56:60-65.
24. Gomes, J. A. C., Colon, A. H., Dhatt, M. S., and Ramption, R. R. 1981. Placement of Swan-Ganz and pacemaker catheters. N. Engl. J. Med. 305:834.

25. Scott, M. L., Webre, D. R., Arens, J. F., and Ochsner, J. L. 1972. Clinical application of a flow-directed balloon-tipped cardiac catheter. Am. Surg. 38:690-696.
26. Foote, G. A., Schabel, S. I., and Hodges, M. 1974. Pulmonary complications of the flow-directed balloon-tipped catheter. N. Engl. J. Med. 290:927-931.
27. Yorra, F. H., Oblath, R., Jaffe, H., Simmons, D. H., and Levy, S. E. 1974. Massive thrombosis associated with use of the Swan-Ganz catheter. Chest 65:682-684.
28. Hoar, P. F., Stone, J. G., Wicks, A. E., Edie, R. N., and Scholes, J. V. 1978. Thrombogenesis associated with Swan-Ganz catheters. Anesthesiology 48:445-447.
29. Hoar, P. F., Wilson, R. M., Mangano, D. T., Avery, G. J., Szarnicki, R. J., and Hill, J. D. 1981. Heparin bonding reduces thrombogenicity of pulmonary artery catheters. N. Engl. J. Med. 305:993-995.
30. Dye, L. E., Segall, P. H., Russel, R. O., Mantle, J. A., Rogers, W. J. and Rackley, C. E. 1978. Deep venous thrombosis of the upper extremity associated with use of the Swan-Ganz catheter. Chest 73:673-675.
31. Chastre, J., Cornud, F., Bouchama, A., Viau, F., Benacerraff, R., and Gilbert, C. 1982. Thrombosis as a complication of pulmonary-artery catheterization via the internal jugular vein. N. Engl. J. Med. 306:278-281.
32. Snow, P. 1980. Swan-Ganz catheter and superior vena cava syndrome. JAMA 243:1525.
33. Richman, K. A., Kim, Y. L., and Marshall, B. E. 1980. Thrombocytopenia and altered platelet kinetics associated with prolonged pulmonary-artery catheterization in the dog. Anesthesiology 53:101-105.
34. Kim, Y. L., Richman, K. A., and Marshall, B. E. 1980. Thrombocytopenia associated with Swan-Ganz catheterization in patients. Anesthesiology 55:261-262.
35. Swedlow, D., Kim, Y., Richman, K. and Marshall, B. 1980. Thrombocytopenia associated with prolonged pulmonary artery catheterization in children. Crit. Care Med. 8(Abstract):273.
36. Goodman, D. J., Rider, A. K., Billingham, M. E., and Schroeder, J. S. 1974. Thromboembolic complications with the indwelling balloon-tipped pulmonary arterial catheter. N. Engl. J. Med. 291:777.
37. McLoud, T. C., and Putman, C. E. 1975. Radiology of the Swan-Ganz catheter and associated pulmonary complications. Radiology 116:19-22.
38. Chun, G. M. H., and Ellstad, M. H. 1971. Perforation of the pulmonary artery by a Swan-Ganz catheter. N. Engl. J. Med. 284:1041-1042.
39. Lapin, E. S., and Murray, J. A. 1972. Hemoptysis with flow-directed cardiac catheterization. JAMA 220:1246.
40. German, J. C., Allyn, P. A., and Bartlett, R. H. 1973. Pulmonary artery pressure monitoring in acute burn management. Arch. Surg. 106:788-791.
41. Golden, M. S., Pinder, T., Anderson, W. T., and Cheitlin, M. D. 1973. Fatal pulmonary hemorrhage complicating use of a flow-directed balloon-tipped catheter in a patient receiving anticoagulant therapy. Am. J. Cardiol. 32:865-867.
42. Lemen, R., Jones, J. G., and Cowan, G. 1975. A mechanism of pulmonary-artery perforation by Swan-Ganz catheters. N. Engl. J. Med. 292:211.
43. Page, D. W., Teres, D., and Hartshorn, J. W. 1974. Fatal hemorrhage from Swan-Ganz catheter. N. Engl. J. Med. 291:260.
44. Shin, B., Ayella, R. J., and McAslan, T. C. 1977. Pitfalls of Swan-Ganz catheterization. Crit. Care Med. 5:125-127.
45. Pape, L. A., Haffejee, C. I., Markis, J. E., Ockene, I. S., Paraskos, J. A., Dalen, J. E., and Alpert, J. S. 1979. Fatal pulmonary hemorrhage after use of the flow-directed balloon-tipped catheter. Ann. Intern. Med. 90:344-347.
46. Rubin, S. A., and Puckett, R. P. 1979. Pulmonary artery-bronchial fistula—A new complication of Swan-Ganz catheterization. Chest 75:515-516.

47. Haapaniemi, J., Gadowski, R., Naini, M., Green, H., MacKenzie, D., and Rubenfire, M. 1979. Massive hemoptysis secondary to flow-directed thermodilution catheters. Cathet. Cardiovasc. Diagn. 5:151-157.
48. Krantz, E. M., and Viljoen, J. R. 1979. Hemoptysis following insertion of a Swan-Ganz catheter. Br. J. Anaesth. 51:457-459.
49. Ohn, K. C., Cottrell, J. E., and Turndorf, H. 1979. Hemoptysis from a pulmonary-artery catheter. Anesthesiology 51:485-486.
50. Deren, M. M., Barash, P. G., Hammond, G. L., and Saieh, T. 1979. Perforation of the pulmonary artery requiring pneumonectomy after the use of a flow-directed (Swan-Ganz) catheter. Thorax 34:550-553.
51. Paulson, D. M., Scott, S. M., and Sethi, G. K. 1980. Pulmonary hemorrhage associated with balloon flotation catheters. J. Thorac. Cardiovasc. Surg. 80:453-458.
52. Rosenbaum, L., Rosenbaum, S. H., Askanazi, J., and Hyman, A. I. 1981. Small amount of hemoptysis as an early warning sign of pulmonary artery rupture by a pulmonary arterial catheter. Crit. Care Med. 9:319-320.
53. Farber, D. L., Rose, D. M., Bassell, G. M., and Eugene, J. 1981. Hemoptysis and pneumothorax after removal of a persistently wedged pulmonary artery catheter. Crit. Care Med. 9:494-495.
54. Kelly, T. F., Morris, G. C., Crawford, E. S., Espada, R., and Howell, J. F. 1981. Perforation of the pulmonary artery with Swan-Ganz catheters. Ann. Surg. 193:686-692.
55. McDaniel, D. D., Stone, J. G., Faltas, A. N., Khambatta, H. J., Thys, D. M., Antunes, A. M., and Bregman, D. 1981. Catheter-induced pulmonary artery hemorrhage. J. Thorac. Cardiovasc. Surg. 82:1-4.
56. Barash, P. G., Nardi, D., Hammond, G., Walker-Smith, G., Capuano, D., Laks, H., Kopriva, C. J., Baue, A. E., and Geha, A. S. 1981. Catheter-induced pulmonary artery perforation. J. Thorac. Cardiovasc. Surg. 82:5-12.
57. Colvin, M. P., Savege, T. M., and Lewis, C. T. 1975. Pulmonary damage from a Swan-Ganz catheter. Br. J. Anaesth. 47:1107-1109.
58. Connors, J. P., Sandza, J. G., Shaw, R. C., Wolff, G. A., and Lombardo, J. A. 1980. Lobar pulmonary hemorrhage—An unusual complication of Swan-Ganz catheterization. Arch. Surg. 115:883-885.
59. Meltzer, R., Kint, P. P., and Simoons, M. 1981. Hemoptysis after flushing Swan-Ganz catheters in the wedge position. N. Engl. J. Med. 304:1171.
60. Swan, H. J. C., and Ganz, W. 1974. Guidelines for use of balloon-tipped catheter. Am. J. Cardiol. 34:119-120.
61. Swan, H. J. C., and Ganz, W. 1979. Complications with flow-directed balloon-tipped catheters. Ann. Intern. Med. 91:494.
62. Carlon, G. C., Howland, W. S., Kahn, R. C., Turnbull, A. D., and Makowsky, M. 1978. Unusual complications during pulmonary artery catheterization. Crit. Care Med. 6:364-365.
63. Gordon, E. P., Quan, S. F., and Schlobohm, R. M. 1980. Hydromediastinum after placement of a thermodilution pulmonary arterial catheter. Anesth. Analg. 59:159-160.
64. Greene, J. F., and Cummings, K. C. 1973. Aseptic thrombotic endocardial vegetations. A complication of indwelling pulmonary artery catheters. JAMA 225:1525-1526.
65. Greene, J. F., Fitzwater, J. E., and Clemmer, T. P. 1975. Septic endocarditis and indwelling pulmonary artery catheters. JAMA 233:891-892.
66. Pace, N. L., and Horton, W. 1975. Indwelling pulmonary artery catheters—Their relationship to aseptic thrombotic endocardial vegetations. JAMA 233:893-894.

67. Smith, W. R., Glauser, F. L., and Jemison, P. 1976. Ruptured chordae of the tricuspid valve. Chest 70:790-792.
68. Ehrie, M., Morgan, A. P., Moore, F. D., and O'Connor, N. E. 1978. Endocarditis with the indwelling balloon-tipped pulmonary artery catheter in burn patients. J. Trauma 18:664-666.
69. O'Toole, J. D., Wurtzbacher, J. J., Wearner, N. E., and Jain, A. C. 1979. Pulmonary-valve injury and insufficiency during pulmonary-artery catheterization. N. Engl. J. Med. 301:1167-1168.
70. Duong, H. D., Warner, O. G., and Sampson, C. C. 1980. Tricuspid valve and papillary muscle avulsion following flow-directed catheter removal. J. Natl. Med. Assoc. 72:703-705.
71. Lipp, H., and Resnekov, L. 1971. Intracardiac knotting of a flow-directed balloon catheter. N. Engl. J. Med. 284:220.
72. Swaroop, S. 1972. Knotting of two central venous monitoring catheters. Am. J. Med. 53:386-388.
73. Daum, S., and Schapira, M. 1973. Intracardiac knot formation in a Swan-Ganz catheter. Anesth. Analg. 52:862-863.
74. Mond, H. G., Clark, D. W., Nesbitt, S. J., and Schlant, R. C. 1975. A technique for unknotting an intracardiac flow-directed balloon catheter. Chest 67:731-733.
75. Dach, J. L., Galbut, D. L., and LePage, J. R. 1981. The knotted Swan-Ganz catheter: New solution to a vexing problem. Am. J. Roentgenol. 137:1274-1275.
76. Meister, S. G., Furr, C. M., Engel, T. R., Sones, M., and Frankl, W. S. 1977. Knotting of a flow-directed catheter about a cardiac structure. Cathet. Cardiovasc. Diagn. 3:171-175.
77. Schwartz, K. V., and Garcia, F. G. 1977. Entanglement of Swan-Ganz catheter around an intracardiac structure. JAMA 237:1198-1199.
78. Fibuch, E. E., and Tuohy, G. F. 1980. Intracardiac knotting of a flow-directed balloon-tipped catheter. Anesth. Analg. 59:217-219.
79. Voci, G., Gazek, F. A., Burris, A. C., and Zatuchni, J. 1980. Retrieval of entrapped and knotted balloon-tipped catheters from the right heart. Ann. Intern. Med. 92:638-639.
80. Kumar, S. P., Yans, J., Kwatra, M., Loesch, D. M., and Viturawong, V. 1980. Removal of a knotted flow-directed catheter by a non-surgical method. Ann. Intern. Med. 92:639-640.
81. Block, P. C. 1976. Snaring of a Swan-Ganz catheter. J. Thorac. Cardiovasc. Surg. 71:917-919.
82. Andreasson, S. E., and Appelgren, L. K. 1979. Complication of Swan-Ganz catheter. Crit. Care Med. 7:256.
83. Applefeld, J. J., Caruthers, T. E., Reno, D. J., and Civetta, J. M. 1978. Assessment of the sterility of long-term cardiac catheterization using the thermodilution Swan-Ganz catheter. Chest 74:377-380.
84. Caruthers, T. E., Reno, D. J., and Civetta, J. M. 1979. Implications of positive blood cultures associated with Swan-Ganz catheters. Crit. Care Med. 7 (Abstract):135.
85. Shaffer, L. J. 1979. Sterility and repositioning of the Swan-Ganz catheter. Chest 75:743.
86. Applefeld, J. J. 1979. Sterility and repositioning of the Swan-Ganz catheter. Chest 75:743.
87. Kopman, E. A., and Sandza, J. G. 1978. Manipulation of the pulmonary-artery catheter after placement: Maintenance of sterility. Anesthesiology 48:373-374.
88. Cerra, F., Milch, R., and Lajos, T. Z. 1973. Pulmonary artery catheterization in critically ill surgical patients. Ann. Surg. 177:37-39.

89. Sorensen, M. B. 1975. Pulmonary artery pressure measurements in surgical patients. Scand. J. Thorac. Cardiovasc. Surg. 9:264-270.
90. Conahan, T. J. 1979. Air embolization during percutaneous Swan-Ganz catheter placement. Anesthesiology 50:360-361.
91. Birrer, R. B., and Plotz, C. M. 1981. Bernard-Horner syndrome associated with Swan-Ganz catheter. N.Y. State J. Med. 81:362-364.
92. McNabb, T. G., Green, L. H., and Parker, F. L. 1975. A potentially serious complication with Swan-Ganz catheter placement by the percutaneous internal jugular route. Br. J. Anesth. 47:895-987.
93. Katz, S. A., and Cohen, E. L. 1975. Urologic complication associated with Swan-Ganz catheter. Urology 6:716-718.
94. Smith, G. B., and Willatts, S. M. 1981. A hazard of Swan-Ganz catheterization. Anaesthesia 36:398-401.
95. Parulkar, D. C., Grundy, E. M., and Bennett, E. J. 1978. Fracture of a float catheter. Br. J. Anaesth. 50:201-203.

Section II

Clinical Applications

Chapter 4

Direct Measurements and Derived Calculations Using the Pulmonary Artery Catheter

Charles L. Sprung, Eric C. Rackow, and Joseph M. Civetta

The pulmonary artery catheter permits the study of the pathophysiology of disease at the bedside. Many physicians decide a patient requires pulmonary artery catheterization, perform the catheterization, and shortly thereafter leave the bedside. Unfortunately, they do not take full advantage of the catheter's potential. Hemodynamic monitoring provides greater diagnostic precision and furnishes a safe means of assessing the results of therapy. An important prerequisite for optimal hemodynamic monitoring is an understanding of normal physiologic measurements and the significance of alterations in different disease states. This Clinical Applications section presents the cardiopulmonary variables that can be measured or calculated with the use of the flotation catheter. In this section, Chapter 5 also analyzes the use of this data in individual patients with typical disease entities requiring catheterization.

The introduction of a pulmonary artery catheter rather than a central venous pressure (CVP) catheter affords a tremendous increase in physiologic information. The catheter measures pulmonary artery systolic, diastolic, and mean pressures, right ventricular filling pressures, pulmonary artery wedge pressures, an estimation of left ventricular filling pressure and left ventricular function, cardiac output, and true mixed venous blood samples.

The following variables are measured or calculated and provide important cardiopulmonary indices (1-4). The cardiopulmonary profile sheet currently used in our critical care unit together with the appropriate calculations are demonstrated in Profile Chart 4.1. Normal values can be seen in Table 4.1.

Profile Chart 4. 1. Cardiopulmonary profile, Miami V. A. Hospital Medical Intensive Care Unit

Patient Name: ______________________

Hospital no.: ______________________

Diagnosis/procedure: ______________________

Enter: Date/time:				
Cardiac output (CO)				
Systolic blood pressure (SBP)				
Diastolic blood pressure (DBP)				
Mean arterial pressure (MAP)				
Heart rate (HR)				
Mean pulmonary artery pressure (MPAP)				
Pulmonary artery wedge pressure (PWP)				
Central venous pressure (CVP)				
Body surface area (BSA)				
Data:				
Stroke volume (SV) (CO/HR)				
Cardiac index (CI) (CO/BSA)				
Stroke index (SI) (SV/BSA)				
Right ventricular stroke work (RVSW) [SI × (MPAP-CVP) × 0.0136]				
RVSW/CVP ratio				
Left ventricular stroke work (LVSW) [SI × (MAP-PWP) × 0.0136]				
LVSW/PWP ratio				
Systemic vascular resistance (SVR) (MAP-CVP/CO) 79.9				
Pulmonary vascular resistance (PVR) (MPAP-PWP/CO) 79.9				

Enter:					
Hemoglobin (Hgb)					
FIO_2					
$PaCO_2$					
PaO_2					
SaO_2					
PvO_2					
SvO_2					
Data:					
Capillary O_2 content (CcO_2) [Hgb × alv O_2 sat × 1.36 + (PaO_2 × 0.003)]					
Mixed venous O_2 content (CvO_2) [Hgb × Ven O_2 sat × 1.36 + (PvO_2 × 0.003)]					
Arterial O_2 content (CaO_2) [Hgb × Art O_2 sat × 1.36 + (PaO_2 × 0.003)]					
Arteriovenous O_2 content difference ($avDO_2$) (CaO_2 - CvO_2)					
O_2 delivery (CO × CaO_2 × 10)					
O_2 consumption (VO_2) (CO × $avDO_2$ × 10)					
O_2 utilization ratio ($avDO_2/CaO_2$)					
Intrapulmonary shunt (Qs/Qt) (CcO_2-CaO_2/CcO_2-CvO_2)					
PaO_2/FIO_2					
Vasopressors or vasodilators (μ/k/m)					
PEEP					
Respirator rate					
Tidal volume					
PIP					

Table 4.1. Normal values

Parameter	Normal value
I. Pressures (mm Hg)	
A. Systemic artery	
1. Peak systolic (SBP)	100-140
2. End diastolic (DBP)	60-90
3. Mean (MAP)	70-105
B. Pulmonary artery wedge (PWP) [for left atrial (LAP)]	
1. Diastolic mean	2-12
2. "a" wave	3-15
C. Pulmonary artery (PA)	
1. Peak systolic (PASP)	15-30
2. End diastolic (PADP)	4-12
3. Mean	9-16
D. Right ventricle (RV)	
1. Peak systolic	15-30
2. End diastolic	0-8
E. Right atrial (RA) or Central venous pressure (CVP) mean	0-8
II. Resistance ($dyne{\cdot}sec{\cdot}cm^{-5}$)	
A. Systemic Vascular Resistance (SVR)	900-1400
B. Pulmonary Vascular Resistance (PVR)	150-250
III. Flows	
A. Cardiac output (CO) (liters/min)	Varies with Size
B. Cardiac index (CI) (liters/min/m^2)	2.8-4.2
C. Stroke index (SI) (ml/min/m^2)	30-65
IV. Heart rate (HR) (beats/min)	60-100
V. Left ventricular stroke work (LVSW) (gram·meters/m^2)	43-61
VI. Right ventricular stroke work (RVSW) (gram·meters/m^2)	7-12
VII. Hemoglobin concentration (g/dl)	12-16
VIII. A. Arterial oxygen tension (PO_2) (mm Hg)	70-100
B. Arterial oxygen saturation (%)	93-98
IX. A. Mixed venous oxygen tension ($P\bar{v}O_2$) (mm Hg)	36-42
B. Mixed venous oxygen saturation (%)	75
X. Arterial-mixed venous oxygen content difference ($avDO_2$) (ml/dl)	3-5
XI. Oxygen delivery (mlO_2/min)	640-1400
XII. Oxygen consumption (VO_2) (mlO_2/min)	180-280
XIII. Oxygen extraction ratio (%)	0.22-0.30
XIV. Pulmonary venous admixture $\frac{(Qs)}{(Qt)}$ (%)	$<$ 3-5

I. DIRECTLY MEASURED VARIABLES

A very important yet not often recognized problem is the actual effect of invasive monitoring on the patient's hemodynamic measurements. It is clear that invasive monitoring changes the patient. Responses during invasive instrumentation have been shown to be significantly different than during a basal state or by noninvasive studies (5). This problem is probably lessened by continuous hemodynamic monitoring over longer periods of time and emphasizes the importance of serial monitoring of parameters rather than relying on an isolated value. To provide continuity, pressures should be recorded with the patient in the same position (usually supine).

A. Heart Rate

The rhythmic dilation of an artery produced by the volume of blood ejected by the cardiac contraction is termed *heart rate* (HR). The heart rate is usually measured by palpation or by the monitored ventricular rate on the electrocardiogram (ECG).

B. Blood Pressure

Blood Pressure (BP) is the tension of blood within a vessel. Arterial blood pressure is a function of left ventricular contraction, resistance and elasticity of arterial walls, viscosity, and blood volume.

1. Systolic BP Systolic BP (SBP) is the pressure occurring at ventricular systole.

2. Diastolic BP Diastolic BP (DBP) is the pressure occurring during ventricular diastole.

Blood pressure can be indirectly measured with a sphygmomanometer or directly measured with an arterial catheter. The indirect method usually underestimates systolic blood pressure and overestimates diastolic pressure by several millimeters of mercury.

3. Mean BP Mean BP (MAP) is calculated by the addition of one-third the pulse pressure (systolic minus diastolic) to the diastolic blood pressure.

Increased pulse pressure may be secondary to cardiac mechanisms (increased stroke volume secondary to bradycardia, anxiety, aortic regurgitation) or peripheral mechanisms secondary to arteriovenous shunts, arteriolar-capillary vasodilation (fever, anemia, hyperthyroidism, cirrhosis, beriberi) or decreased distensibility of arterial vessels (atherosclerosis or hypertension). Decreased pulse pressure may be related to decreased left ventricular ejection rate or volume (shock, heart failure, hypovolemia), peripheral vasoconstriction (shock, hypovolemia, vasoconstricting drugs), and mechanical causes (aortic or mitral valve obstruction).

C. Cardiac Output

Cardiac output (CO) is the volume of blood pumped by the heart. The function of the heart as a pump is determined by four factors: preload, myocardial contractility, afterload, and heart rate. The cardiac output is usually determined by the thermodilution method available with the pulmonary artery catheter but other methods (Fick or green dye indicator-dilution method) are available. Normal cardiac output varies with age decreasing from approximately 4.5 liters/min/m^2 at age 7 to 2.5 liters/min/m^2 at age 70.

*1. **Preload*** Ventricular preload is the end-diastolic stretch of the muscle fiber which, in the intact ventricle, is the end-diastolic volume.

Cardiac responsiveness has been shown to be related to the presystolic fiber length. Left ventricular "Starling curves" can be constructed by plotting left ventricular work or stroke volume as a function of left ventricular myocardial fiber length (Figure 4.1). It is interesting that a majority of Starling's original experiments were performed using right-sided venous pressures (6). He did, however, note an increase in left auricular pressures as central venous pressure (CVP) increased and as output from both ventricles increased (6). Because the end-diastolic fiber length and intraventricular pressure are usually related, it has become commonplace in clinical circumstances to measure left ventricular end-diastolic pressure, pulmonary artery wedge pressure (PWP), or pulmonary artery diastolic pressure, which are more easily measured, rather than fiber length or left ventricular volume, which are not easily obtainable. Therefore, a Starling curve can be constructed for an individual patient by performing serial cardiac output determinations and correlating cardiac output, stroke volume, or stroke work with different hydrostatic filling pressures. As one increases pulmonary artery wedge pressure with volume resuscitation, one would expect to see an increase in stroke volume or stroke work (Figure 4.2). Under normal condi-

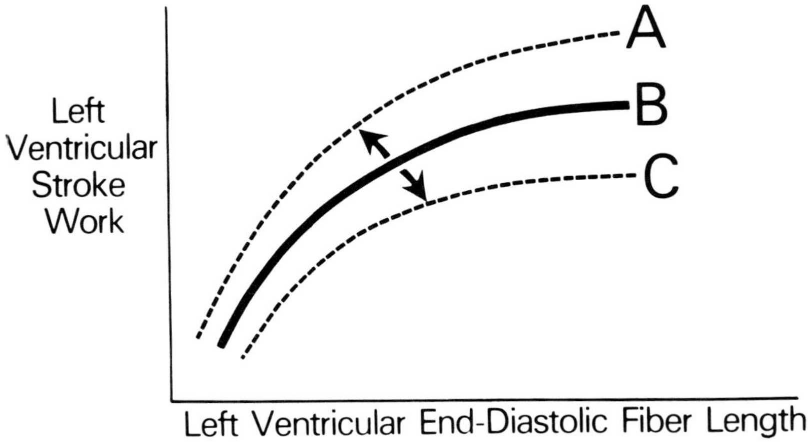

Figure 4.1. The effect of the myocardial contractile state on the left ventricular stroke work at a given left ventricular end-diastolic fiber length or volume. Curve B is the normal curve. Curve A represents a shift to the left associated with increased contractility; whereas curve C demonstrates a shift to the right associated with decreased contractility.

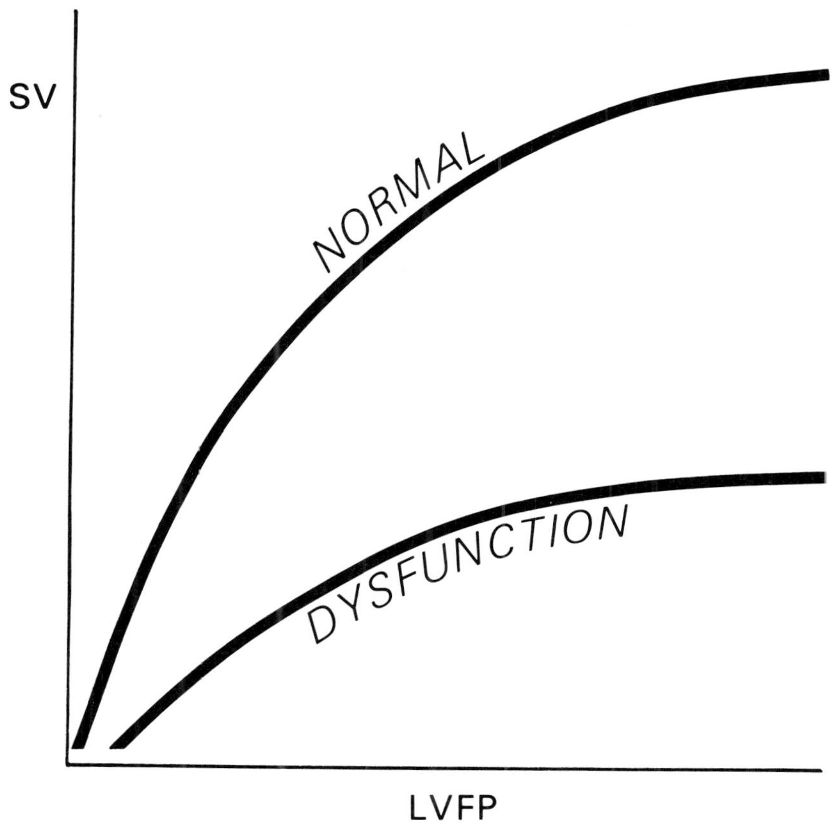

Figure 4.2. A Frank-Starling curve demonstrating the relationship between left ventricular filling pressure and stroke volume. In the face of myocardial dysfunction stroke volume can still increase with increasing left ventricular filling pressure. The curve, however, is much flatter than the normal curve and a lesser stroke volume is produced for a similar left ventricular filling pressure.

tions, small increases in filling pressure are associated with significant increases in cardiac performance. The importance of initial fiber length rather than intraventricular pressure is accepted. Therefore, despite the fact that these two factors are usually related, the relation may vary considerably because of changes in ventricular compliance or changes within the pericardium or thorax. These changes may not be recognized by measurements performed with the pulmonary artery catheter as pulmonary artery wedge pressure may not correlate with left ventricular end-diastolic volume but may have clinical significance as an indicator of pulmonary edema (Figure 4.3) (7).

The three factors which influence preload are blood volume, the distribution of the blood volume (related to venous tone and intrathoracic pressure), and atrial contraction.

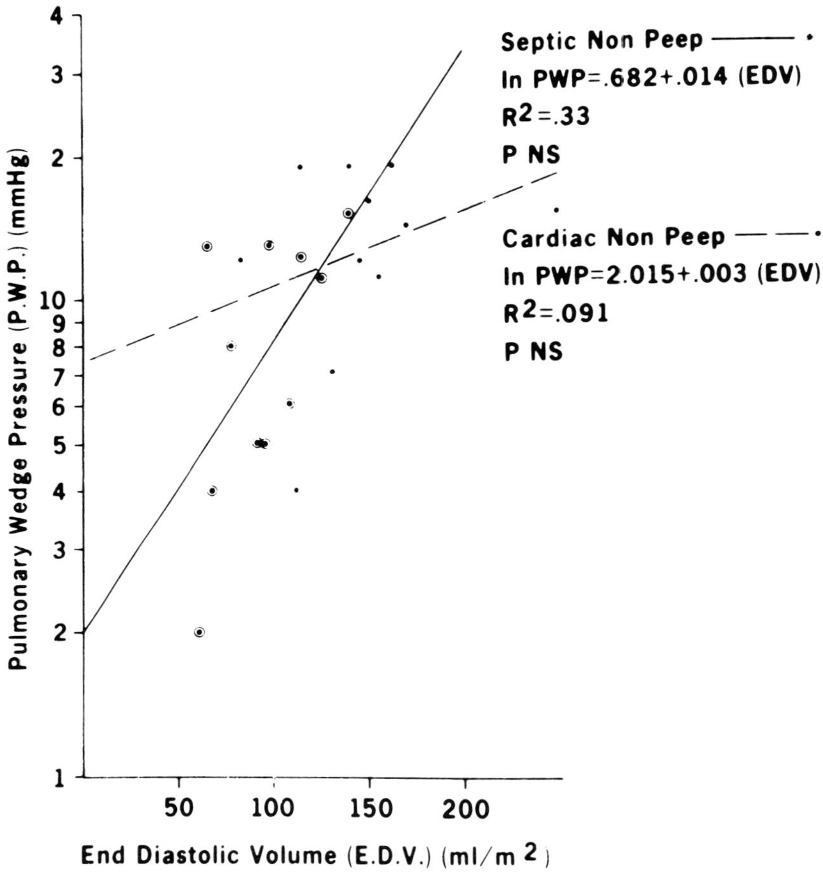

Figure 4.3. The demonstration of the lack of correlation between left ventricular end-diastolic volume and the pulmonary artery wedge pressure in both cardiac and noncardiac groups of patients. Reproduced from Calvin et al., 1981 (7) with permission.

2. Contractility Contractility refers to a change in the velocity of muscle shortening at any tension level and to changes in the maximum velocity of shortening extrapolated to zero load. A change in the inotropic state of the muscle occurs without a change in the fiber length (end-diastolic volume). In the heart, a change in contractility denotes a change independent of preload or afterload. Inotropic agents such as digitalis, calcium, or catecholamines increase contractility by increasing the velocity of shortening of the muscle at zero load. An increase in contractility is associated with an increase in stroke volume or stroke work despite no change in preload. This moves the ventricular Starling curve upward and to the left (See Figures 4.1 and 4.2). A decrease in contractility causes a shift downward and to the right resulting in a lower stroke volume or stroke work at the same filling conditions (Figure 4.1). Increases in contractility are therefore associated with increases in cardiac output, whereas decreases in contractility are associated with a decreased cardiac output. It is evident, therefore, that contractility is dependent on several factors, including circulating catecholamines, pharmacologic inotropes (digitalis, isoproterenol) and depressants (procainamide, barbiturates), physiologic depressants, (acidosis, hypoxia), and a loss of myocardium (myocardial infarction).

3. Afterload Afterload is the tension that develops in the ventricular wall during systole. The tension is influenced by intraventricular pressure (or aortic pressure), ventricular radius, ventricular wall thickness, aortic compliance, peripheral vascular resistance, and the mass and viscosity of blood. Afterload increases with increased pressure (hypertension), an enlarged ventricle (congestive heart failure), a thin ventricular wall, increased resistance, and increased blood viscosity. Decreases in afterload occur with peripheral or central shunting of blood (arteriovenous fistula, cirrhosis, sepsis, patent ductus arteriosus), vasodilation (hyperthermia, thyrotoxicosis), or reduced blood viscosity (anemia).

4. Heart Rate The cardiac output is equal to the product of the stroke volume and heart rate. Therefore, an increase in heart rate is one of the most simple and effective means of increasing cardiac output. An increase in pulse may increase cardiac output significantly only up to a certain rate. Above this rate (170-180 beats/min for young normal individuals, 120-140 beats/min for older people or patients with heart disease) cardiac output may fall. This is related to the decreased time of diastole, which limits ventricular filling and coronary blood flow. It should also be noted that an increase in heart rate may also increase cardiac output by an increase in ventricular contractility (8).

For the above reasons, an increased cardiac output is found in thyrotoxicosis, arteriovenous fistula, sepsis, hyperthermia, anemia, and beriberi. A decreased cardiac output is noted in disease states with decreased contracting muscle mass (infarction or ischemia), cardiac arrhythmias, mechanical defects (ventricular septal defect, mitral insufficiency), hypovolemia, increased vascular resistance, and metabolic conditions.

D. Central Venous Pressure

Up to the advent of the pulmonary artery catheter, the central venous pressure (CVP) was used extensively in the treatment of critically ill patients. Right atrial pressure is equal to the right ventricular diastolic pressure and CVP. Implicit in the use of CVP monitoring is the assumption that right ventricular function parallels left ventricular function. Central venous pressure, however, is influenced not only by ventricular function and compliance, but also by intravascular volume, venous return, systemic venous tone, and pulmonary vascular resistance. CVP may not increase until right ventricular end-diastolic pressure rises. Therefore, left ventricular failure and pulmonary congestion may be present with normal CVP.

The central venous pressure has been shown to have little relationship to left atrial or pulmonary artery wedge pressure (PWP) in patients with valvular heart disease (9, 10), coronary artery disease (11, 12), or pulmonary hypertension (13). Mangano (14) noted that if the relationship between CVP and PWP is examined in individual patients with coronary artery disease rather than in an entire patient population, correlations are good in patients with ejection fractions greater than 0.5 and without areas of dyssynergy by angiocardiography. Patients with left ventricular dyssynergy and ejection fractions less than 0.4 had poor correlations (14). In patients with acute myocardial infarction, CVP correlated poorly with PWP and with roentgenographic evidence of left ventricular failure (Figure 4.4) (15). In the absence of cardiopulmonary disease, CVP remains a reliable indicator of right- and left-sided pressures (11), but the correlation may not be striking ($r = 0.68$) (16). The assumption that CVP correlates well with left ventricular function is not valid in the critically ill patient (11, 17) and CVP does not correlate with PWP (Figure 4.5). Finally, diuresis and volume resuscitation cause directional changes in CVP which often reflect similar changes in PWP (11, 12, 15, 17, 18). Unfortunately, on many occasions there is an opposite or lack of change in CVP compared to the change in PWP. Therefore, it is not surprising that the pulmonary artery catheter has replaced the CVP for hemodynamic monitoring in many instances. The CVP may still have an important role in initial volume resuscitation, right ventricular infarction, and cardiac tamponade. The CVP is increased in patients with right ventricular failure and/or infarction, tricuspid regurgitation, pericardial tamponade, and hypervolemia. The CVP is usually decreased in patients with hypovolemia. Clues to the diagnosis of tricuspid insufficiency and pericardial tamponade can be made by inspecting the wave forms. The presence of "giant V waves" in the right atrial tracing is indicative of tricuspid insufficiency. Diastolic pressures of the right atrium, right ventricle, pulmonary artery, and pulmonary capillaries are equal and of similar contour in pericardial tamponade.

E. Pulmonary Artery Pressures

Pulmonary artery systolic (PASP), diastolic (PADP), mean (MPAP), and pulmonary artery wedge pressure can be measured with the balloon-tipped flotation catheter. Pulmonary artery pressure is equal to right ventricular pressure during systole when the pulmonary valve is open. The initial enthusiasm for catheterization of the pulmonary artery was based on the realization that a properly constituted pressure monitoring system could use pulmonary pressures to reflect left ventricular filling pressures. For this measurement to be accurate, a specific configuration of the vasculature distal to the catheter tip must be envisioned and physiologically possible. The principles of the physics describing flow and pressure in any system recognize that flow can only be created if there is a pressure differential at the beginning and at the end of a tubular system. If there is no pressure differen-

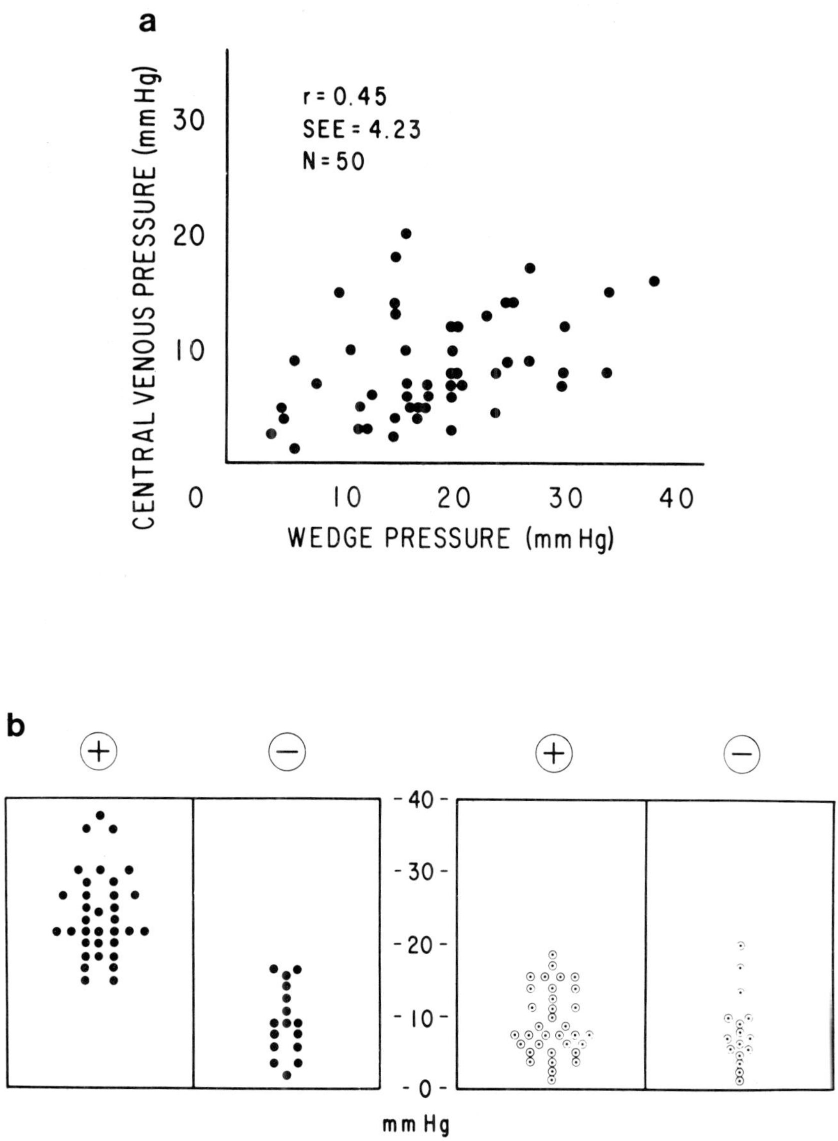

Figure 4.4. *a*, The poor correlation between simultaneously measured central venous pressure and pulmonary artery wedge pressure in patients with acute myocardial infarction. *b*, The correlation between pulmonary artery wedge pressure (solid circles) and central venous pressure (open circles) and the presence (+) or absence (-) of radiologic pulmonary congestion. A PWP of 18 mm Hg provided an excellent separation of the two radiologic groups. CVP, on the other hand, could not separate the two groups. Reproduced from Forrester et al., 1971 (15) with permission.

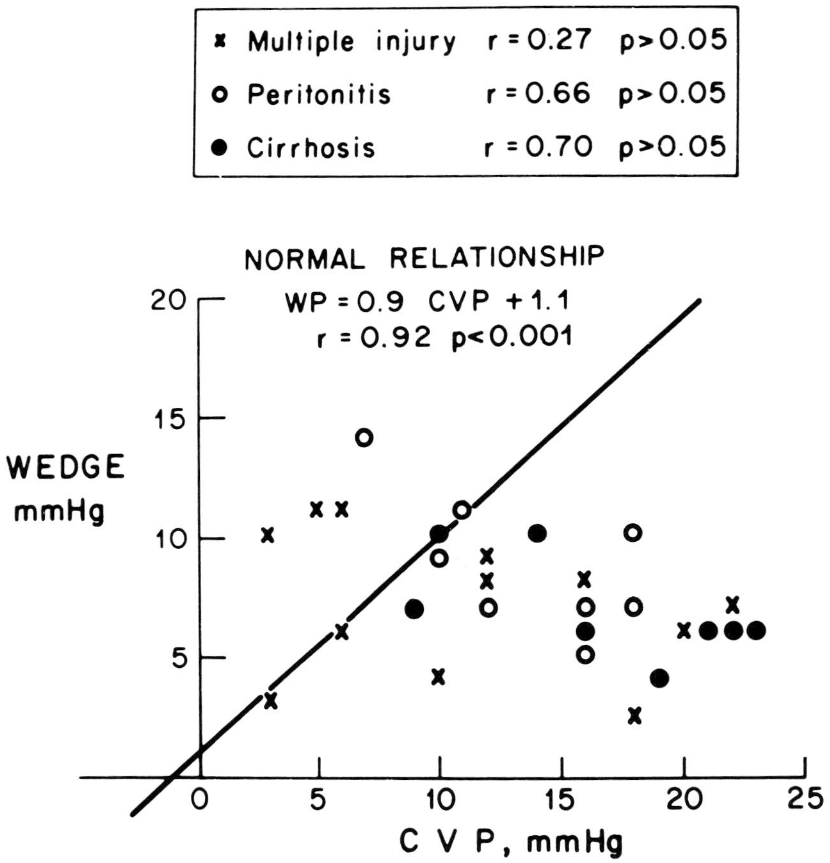

Figure 4.5. A comparison of central venous pressure and pulmonary artery wedge pressure in normal patients and those with severe multisystem injury, decompensated cirrhosis, and peritonitis. As opposed to the good relationship in normals, poor relationships are noted in these three disease states. Reproduced from Civetta and Gabel, 1972 (11) with permission.

tial, flow must be absent and the system is in a stagnant state (Figure 4.6). Using this principle in reverse, if one could create a stagnant system in which no forward flow was present, measurement of a distal pressure would be possible and accurate from a proximal source. According to the anatomy involved, the catheter is positioned in a moderately sized pulmonary artery connected to pulmonary arterioles, which in turn lead to the pulmonary capillaries. This anatomic linkage continues through small pulmonary venules and these join together to form the major pulmonary veins. Finally, the pulmonary veins enter the left atrium. On the one hand, this is a complex system; but if no flow is present, pressure measured throughout the system should be constant. In fact, simultaneous left heart and pulmonary artery pressures in man have validated this principle.

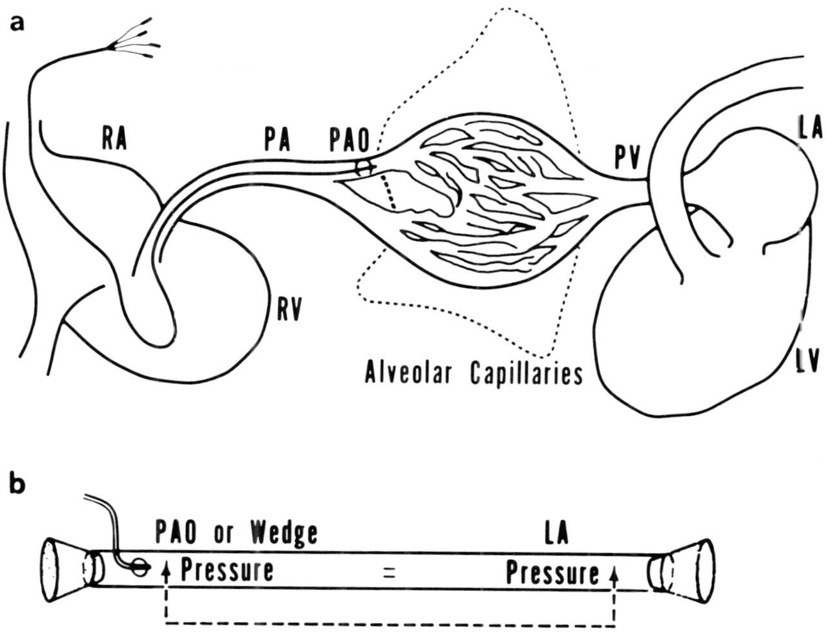

Figure 4.6. Diagramatic representation of a pulmonary artery catheter in the correct position. Note that although the tip of the catheter lies in a pulmonary artery, with the balloon inflated, no flow exists in the system and that the "closed pipe" analogy necessitates equal pressure readings throughout the system.

1. Pulmonary Artery Wedge Pressure (PWP): Pulmonary Capillary Pressure (PCP) or Pulmonary Artery Occlusion Pressure (PAOP) Hellems et al. (19) were the first to demonstrate that the distal opening of a cardiac catheter, wedged into a small branch of a pulmonary artery until the vessel was occluded, formed a free communication with the pulmonary capillaries and veins. Lagerlof and Werko (20) demonstrated that the phasic pressure variations obtained under these circumstances are similar to left atrial pressure curves. Pulmonary artery wedge pressures obtained with a balloon-tipped flotation catheter are identical to those obtained by the standard Cournand catheter (21). Ordinary pulmonary artery catheters without a balloon tip must be manually advanced to measure PWP and then withdrawn, whereas the flotation catheter requires only intermittent inflation of the balloon allowing blood flow to pull the catheter tip into the wedge position. Therefore, catheter manipulation is avoided and long-term monitoring is practical.

Various criteria have been used to verify a true wedge position (22-25).

a. A characteristic waveform. The typical pulmonary artery pressure tracing disappears when the balloon is inflated and reappears promptly after deflation. A distinct, triphasic auricular waveform may not be seen with flotation catheters. Damped pulmonary artery pressure tracings should not be used.

b. A mean PWP lower than MPAP and lower than or equal to PADP.

c. A continuous flush system or free-falling column of fluid to exclude catheter obstruction.

d. Blood withdrawn through the wedge catheter should be fully saturated with oxygen. This blood has a significantly higher pH and arterial oxygen tension (pO_2) and a lower arterial carbon dioxide tension (pCO_2) than simultaneously measured systemic arterial blood (26). This is due to the fact that a wedged catheter obstructs flow to its corresponding lung segment and produces a localized area of high ventilation-perfusion ratio. Blood withdrawn from atelectatic areas of the lung would not be subject to this artifact because equilibration with alveolar gas is prevented. On the other hand, pulmonary capillary blood is fully saturated, even in cases of cyanotic congenital heart disease and in cases with impaired oxygen diffusion, despite peripheral desaturation. This occurs because stasis in the wedged area permits sufficiently longer contact of capillary blood with alveolar air to result in full saturation. Unfortunately, wedged catheter samples may not be fully saturated with oxygen in patients with pulmonary shunts and during positive end-expiratory pressure. Therefore, this criterion may not always apply, despite the fact that some authors consider it the single most essential criterion of validity (22).

In most clinical situations the first three criteria are used together with roentgenographic evidence of proper catheter position. Wedged blood samples may be helpful if one is uncertain of the correct position of the catheter.

An understanding of the importance of the PWP is dependent upon its relationship to left ventricular pressures. In the absence of cardiovascular disease, pulmonary pressures bear a relationship to left ventricular filling pressures; at end-diastole, pressures in the pulmonary artery, left atrium, and left ventricle are equal (27-29). Patients with coronary artery disease and valvular disorders have been shown to have significant correlations between PWP and left atrial pressure (LAP) (21, 23, 30-32). Lappas et al. (23) made 161 measurements in 18 cardiac-surgical patients. The correlations over a wide range of pressures are demonstrated in Figure 4.7. In only 11% were the PWP-LAP differences greater than $\pm$ 1 mm Hg and most of these were $\pm$ 2 mm Hg. Epps and Adler (30) noted equal PWP and LAP in all their patients with mitral stenosis. In a study of 700 patients with assorted cardiac abnormalities, Walston and Kendall (32) noted good correlations between PWP and LAP but the degree of scatter increased as the PWP and LAP rose (Figure 4.8). At PWP below 25 mm Hg there were no significant differences between PWP and LAP. Patients with PWP greater than 25 mm Hg had significant differences between PWP and LAP. The error in predicting LAP

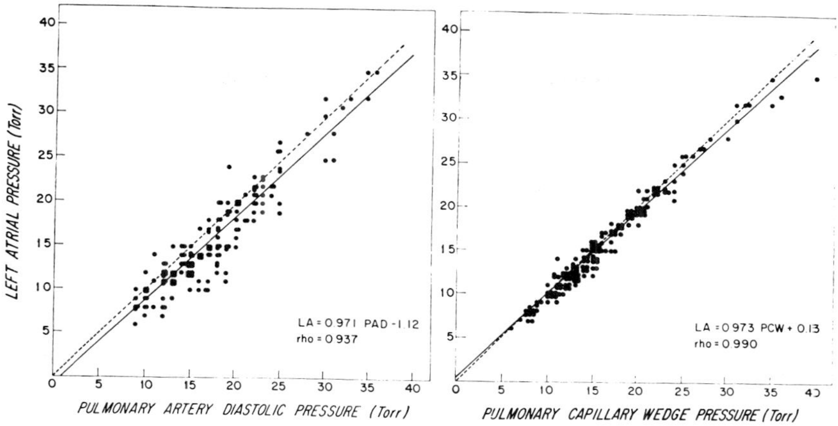

Figure 4.7. The relationship of pulmonary artery diastolic and pulmonary artery wedge pressure to left atrial pressure in cardiac-surgical patients. The correlations are extremely good; PWP correlations are better than PADP. Reproduced from Lappas et al., 1973 (23) with permission.

from PWP was only $\pm$ 2 mm Hg for PWP $\leq$ 10 mm Hg, whereas the error increased with increasing PWP.

Despite the good correlation between PWP and LAP, the relationship between PWP and left ventricular end-diastolic pressure (LVEDP) is not always this close. Before the use of the bedside Swan-Ganz catheter, Sapru et al. (33) noted a close correlation between PWP and LVEDP over a wide range of pressures at rest and after exercise in normal patients and in patients with left ventricular enlargement. They postulated that these close relationships would not occur in the presence of obstructive airway disease, mitral regurgitation, and when atrial systole produces a large pressure pulse. Subsequently, Rahimtoola et al. (34) demonstrated that atrial contraction made a large contribution to left ventricular filling pressures in patients with acute myocardial infarction and that PWP did not accurately reflect LVEDP. The atrial contribution to LVEDP and the difference between PWP and LVEDP was especially large if the LVEDP was greater than 12 mm Hg. Therefore, in patients with left ventricular dysfunction, an elevated LVEDP helps to maintain the force of ventricular contraction. If the LAP and PWP increased commensurate with the LVEDP, the patient would be at risk for the development of pulmonary edema. Left atrial contraction is capable of increasing LVEDP without a proportionate increase in LAP or PWP, thereby dissociating the pulmonary circulation from the consequences of an increased LVEDP (34). Fisher et al. (35) noted significant correlations between PWP and LVEDP during diagnostic cardiac catheterization, but differences of 5 mm Hg or more occurred in more than half the observations secondary to large left ventricular "a" waves. The pulmonary capillary "a"

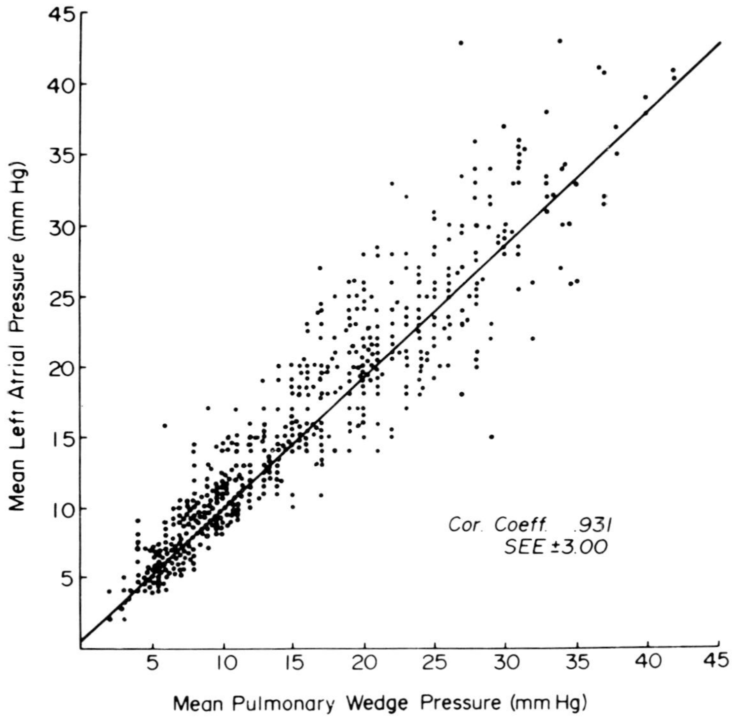

Figure 4.8. The relation between pulmonary artery wedge pressure and left atrial pressure in patients with various cardiac abnormalities. Good correlations are noted. Reproduced from Walston and Kendall, 1973 (32) with permission.

wave pressures correlated best with the LVEDP. In both the Rahimtoola and Fisher studies, the PWP did correlate well with the left ventricular diastolic pressure pre-a. Therefore, in patients with significant atrial contribution to ventricular filling, with mitral valve closure commencing prior to ventricular systole, or with reduced left ventricular compliance, left ventricular end-diastolic pressure may be greater than left ventricular diastolic pressure (LVDP) or PWP.

In summary, PWP correlates well with LAP and LVDP (pre-a) but may not adequately reflect LVEDP. The importance of left ventricular end-diastolic volume (LVEDV) or LVEDP as a reflection of myocardial fiber length and the effects of compliance must be recognized. Therefore, the PWP may not be the best reflection of myocardial fiber length and may not be ideal for the construction of "Starling curves." The PWP is the most accessible parameter for this purpose, however, and increases in PWP usually do reflect increases in left ventricular volume. The PWP certainly remains a good indicator of pulmonary venous hypertension and pulmonary edema.

Mechanical ventilation and positive end-expiratory pressure (PEEP) can affect the measured intravascular pressures. Increasing levels of PEEP have been shown to decrease cardiac output and increase CVP, MPAP, PWP, and pleural pressure (36-46). Pressures measured in the intrathoracic blood vessels must be related to pleural pressure which rises above atmospheric pressure when PEEP is applied. Under these conditions, atmospheric intravascular pressures may be elevated despite low transmural pressures (intravascular pressures minus intrapleural pressures). Therefore, pressures which appear normal or increased may in fact be inadequate to maintain ventricular filling pressure and perfusion.

Although the PWP typically increases with increasing PEEP (36-39, 41-45), some reports have demonstrated a decrease (38, 40) or no change in PWP (40, 47-49). The studies that noted decreasing PWP with PEEP reported transmural pressures rather than atmospheric pressures (38, 40). Qvist et al. (38) showed that atmospheric PWP increased as concomitant transmural PWP decreased.

As noted in the previous section, the PWP accurately reflects the LAP under most circumstances. There are studies which demonstrate a good correlation between PWP and LAP or LVEDP even during PEEP (37, 42, 43, 45, 46, 50-53), whereas other investigations have noted significant differences between PWP and LAP, LVEDP, or LVEDV under these circumstances (36, 37, 41, 44, 46, 49). Differences in catheter position, type of ventilation, level of PEEP, LAP, therapeutic modalities, and the presence of normal or diseased lungs may have contributed to the dissimilar findings observed in these studies. Those studies which did reveal differences between PWP and LAP typically used 10 cm H_2O of PEEP or more, usually 15-20 cm H_2O (36, 37, 41, 44, 46, 49). Lozman et al. (37) and Jardin et al. (46), for instance, noted that PWP reflected LAP or LVEDP at PEEP levels less than 10 cm H_2O but that PWP did not correlate with LAP or LVEDP when 10 cm H_2O PEEP or more was used. Interestingly, Jardin et al. (46) demonstrated that right atrial pressure correlated well with LVEDP in patients receiving more than 10 cm H_2O of PEEP (Figure 4.9).

The measurement of LAP by PWP requires a fluid-filled segment present from the tip of the catheter until the left atrium. If any part of the pulmonary vasculature distal to the catheter tip is occluded or emptied of blood, the PWP is no longer determined by LAP. Whether the pulmonary capillaries or veins contain blood is a function of pulmonary artery pressure, alveolar pressure, LAP, and the hydrostatic relationships to the left atrium (50). The pressures measured by the balloon-tipped flotation catheter are related to these mechanical forces inside and outside the pulmonary blood vessels. West's zone model (54) displays the importance of these forces and is illustrated in Figure 4.10 (51). The top of the lung is in zone 1 and the

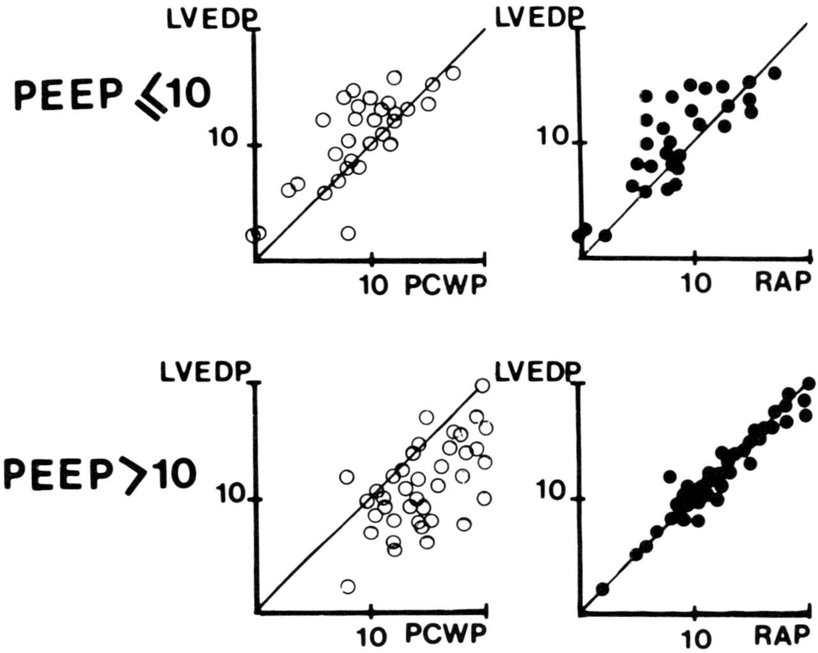

Figure 4.9. The relationship between pulmonary artery wedge pressure (PCWP) or right atrial pressure (RAP) and left ventricular end-diastolic pressure (LVEDP) with positive end-expiratory pressure (PEEP) $\leqslant$ 10 cm H_2O *(upper panel)* and $>$ 10 cm H_2O *(lower panel)*. At a PEEP of 10 cm H_2O or lower, PCWP reflects LVEDP ($r = 0.82$) which is usually higher than RAP ($r = 0.71$). At a PEEP higher than 10 cm H_2O, PCWP is higher than LVEDP ($r = 0.84$), whereas LVEDP bears a close and linear relation to RAP ($r = 0.99$). Reproduced from Jardin et al., 1981 (46) with permission.

pulmonary microvasculature is compressed because alveolar pressure is greater than both pulmonary artery and pulmonary venous pressures. No perfusion occurs in zone 1. The center of the lung is in zone 2 because alveolar pressure is greater than pulmonary venous pressure but less than pulmonary artery pressure. The bottom of the lung is in zone 3 as pulmonary artery and venous pressures are greater than alveolar pressure. In zone 3 a fluid-filled segment of vasculature remains patent without compression. Therefore, for PWP to accurately reflect LAP, alveolar pressure should not exceed pulmonary venous pressure and zone 3 conditions should be fulfilled. If not, airway pressure is transmitted to the collapsible portions of the pulmonary vasculature producing a "Starling resistor" or "vascular waterfall" effect.

In supine animals and humans most of the lung is found in zone 3. Alveolar pressure might be expected to exceed pulmonary venous pressure under conditions of high alveolar pressure (PEEP), low pulmonary venous pressure (hypovolemia), or catheter tip position high in the vertical gradient

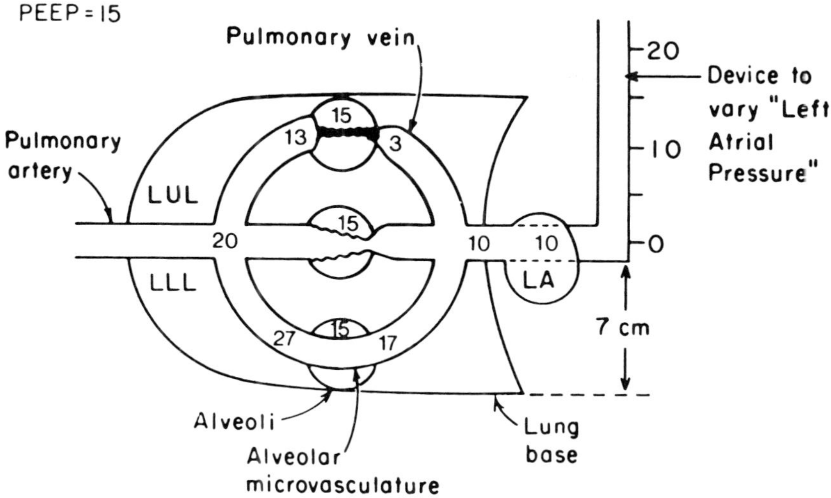

Figure 4.10. A representation of a lung in the supine position with representative vascular and alveolar pressures during PEEP with reference to the vertical height of the lung. At 15 cm H_2O PEEP, vascular pressures vary and are depending on their relative vertical position. LUL, left upper lobe; LLL, left lower lobe; LA, left atrium. Reproduced from Tooker et al., 1978 (51) with permission.

of the lung (above the left atrium). In these situations an increase in zone 2 occurs at the expense of the amount of lung in zone 3. Based on these facts, it is not surprising that every study that investigated catheter position noted that PWP correlated well with LAP if zone 3 criteria were fulfilled (43, 45, 47, 50-53). If the pulmonary artery catheter tip was below the left atrium, PWP correlated with LAP, whereas PWP did not correlate with LAP if the tip was above the left atrium (43, 45, 47, 51-53) (Figures 4.11 and 4.12). Neville demonstrated that PWP did not reflect LAP even if the catheter tip was below the left atrium if PEEP was used in the face of a low LAP (50). In addition, volume expansion and an increase in LAP has been shown to produce a good PWP-LAP correlation even if the catheter tip is above the left atrium (47).

If the position of the catheter is important, how often is a pulmonary artery catheter placed in zone 3? Cross et al. (55) noted that all 35 catheter tips were inserted at or below the mid-heart position and Kronberg et al. (56) demonstrated that 29 of 30 catheters were placed at or vertically below the left atrium. On the other hand, Orta et al. (57) noted that 8 of 18 catheters (44%) were in zone 1 or 2 and Shasby et al. (53) demonstrated that 6 of 30 catheter tips (20%) were located above the left atrium. Unfortunately, zone 3 criteria may not be satisfied even when the catheter tip is at the level of the left atrium when PEEP is used (53). Therefore, it may be extremely difficult to determine that zone 3 conditions exist in clinical situations. Based on the

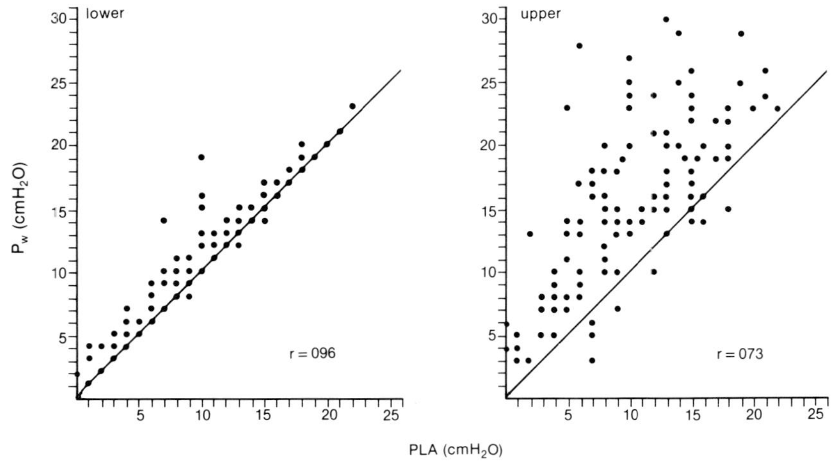

Figure 4.11. A comparison of left atrial pressure (PLA) with lower pulmonary artery wedge pressure (P_w) 4 cm below the atrium and upper P_w 3 cm above the atrium in normal dog lungs at all levels of PEEP within the range of 0 to 30 cm H_2O. The lower P_w correlates well with PLA, whereas the upper P_w overestimates the PLA. Reproduced from Tooker et al., 1978 (51) with permission.

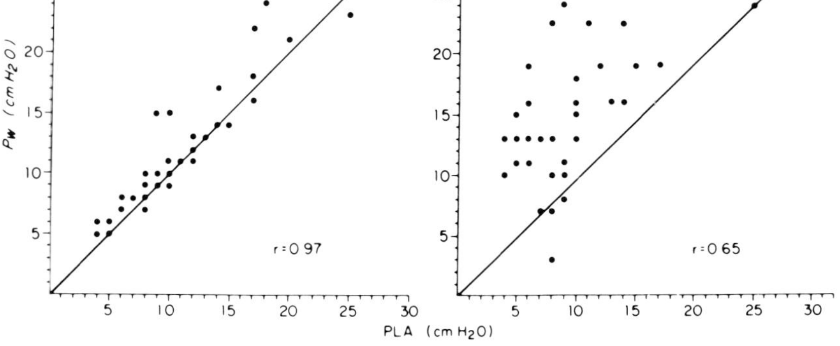

Figure 4.12. A comparison of left atrial pressure (PLA) with lower pulmonary artery wedge pressure (P_w) and upper P_w in dogs with oleic acid induced pulmonary edema at levels of PEEP from 0 to 30 cm H_2O. Again a good correlation in the lower P_w with the PLA in not only normal (Figure 4.11) but injured lungs. Reproduced from Tooker et al., 1978 (51) with permission.

aforementioned data, however, it seems well advised to perform a lateral chest roentgenograph on patients requiring positive pressure ventilation. The vertical level of the pulmonary artery catheter tip can thereby be determined and the "reliability" of the PWP ascertained.

The discontinuation of PEEP constitutes a potential method to validate the PWP as an estimate of LAP and to avoid the possible discrepancies caused by PEEP. Davison et al. (48) found insignificant changes in PWP upon discontinuing PEEP. In no instance was a variation present that could have led to an erroneous appraisal of the hemodynamic status of a patient. One must remember that when PEEP is discontinued, significant decreases in arterial oxygen tensions may occur within minutes. Therefore, the discontinuation of PEEP may be dangerous, and some authors have recommended against this practice (48, 53). In addition, when the effect of PEEP is removed, the hemodynamic status and PWP may be altered secondary to the increase in venous return, pulmonary congestion, and changes in left ventricular function. If there are differences in PWP, one must wonder which PWP (on or off PEEP) is the true reflection of LAP and what is the significance of a PWP off PEEP when PEEP is maintained for 99% of the time? On the other hand, we have noted that significant differences in PWP may occur in patients when PEEP is discontinued. Occasionally profound hypovolemia may be detected by removing PEEP. If a physician believes that the PWP should be measured off PEEP, he or she should attempt to measure the PWP when PEEP is discontinued for other reasons (suctioning), and increased concentrations of oxygen should be given before and after PEEP is stopped. Patients receiving high levels of PEEP and/or patients whose condition deteriorates (bradycardia, hypotension) when PEEP is discontinued should not have PEEP discontinued for PWP measurements.

Various formulas have been developed to determine the effect of PEEP on PWP and thereby obviate the need to discontinue PEEP. Unfortunately, lung compliance and the effects of PEEP will differ from patient to patient and these formulas may not be reliable. In addition, transmural pressures may be calculated by measuring intrapleural pressures using an esophageal balloon or intrapleural catheter. Unfortunately, esophageal pressures may not accurately reflect the nonuniform pressures exerted by the lung on the outside of the heart during PEEP therapy. The risks of intrapleural pressure measurements must be weighed against the value of the information to be gained. Most centers do not therefore measure intrapleural pressures routinely.

Pulmonary artery wedge pressures have been noted to be elevated in many patients with chronic pulmonary disease (58, 59). The magnitude of changes in esophageal pressure during respiratory fluctuation has been shown to correlate well with the changes in PWP (59, 60). Therefore, the increased PWP in these patients may not always represent elevated left ventricular pressures. Several sources of error in the measurement of PWP in patients with chronic pulmonary disorders are present. An increase in the bronchopulmonary venous system which normally connects pulmonary capillaries and peribronchial venules might increase PWP. In addition, increased alveolar pressure due to airway obstruction might interrupt the static column of blood distal to the wedge catheter. However, the increased intrathoracic pressure and pulmonary venous pressure might prevent capillary collapse. Finally, an increase in intrathoracic pressure may be reflected by a rise in pressure in the intrathoracic blood vessels. An increased PWP may therefore be related to elevated intrathoracic pressures rather than left ventricular failure. Despite these reservations, the PWP has been demonstrated to have a good correlation with the LAP (58) and LVEDP (59) in these patients. In a study comparing mean PWP (atmospheric) with effective PWP (atmospheric PWP minus the esophageal pressure) in patients with chronic obstructive pulmonary disease, Rice et al. (60) noted that the differences between the effective and mean PWP were 0.5 ± 1.6 mm Hg (range $\pm$ 3 mm Hg) in all patients when intrathoracic changes were less than 20 mm Hg. Three patients with intrathoracic pressure changes greater than 20 mm Hg had mean PWPs that were much higher than effective PWP. Under these circumstances, absolute PWP may not be very helpful and the risks of catheterization may outweigh the benefits.

PWP is usually taken as the average of several heartbeats at end-expiration with the transducer at the mid-axillary line. PWP is elevated in congestive heart failure, pulmonary venous obstruction, valvular heart disease, and too rapid or too much fluid administration. PWP is low in hypovolemic states.

2. Pulmonary Artery Diastolic or End-Diastolic Pressure (PADP, PAEDP) Pulmonary artery diastolic pressures have also been used to reflect PWP and left ventricular filling pressures. PADP reflects PWP with reasonable accuracy in normal patients and in patients with left ventricular dysfunction, acute myocardial infarction, and chronic lung disease provided severe pulmonary vascular changes are not present (27, 34, 61). PADP has also been found to correlate well with LAP in patients with and without heart disease when pulmonary vascular resistance is normal (23, 28, 31, 62-65). PADP is usually 1-2 mm Hg higher than the PWP and LAP. Despite the correlation, there have been marked differences in individual paired values in some studies, especially in the face of pulmonary hypertension (28, 31, 63). Patients with previous pulmonary disorders and increased pulmonary vascular resistance had no correlation between PADP and LAP or PADP and PWP (61, 62). Therefore, estimation of LAP from PADP is unlikely to be accurate when pulmonary vascular resistance is abnormally elevated. Serial changes in PADP did not predict directional changes of LAP in a group of patients undergoing open heart surgery (64), but did predict directional changes in another group of patients with acute and chronic heart disease, even in those patients with poor baseline correlations (28). PWP has always found to be superior to PADP in estimating the LAP (23, 31, 65). Increased PADP and the difference between the PADP and PWP may be helpful in determining the degree of pulmonary vascular resistance (61, 62). A PADP-PWP difference of 4 to 5 mm Hg can be used as an index to differentiate normal and increased pulmonary vascular resistance (61).

As noted for the PWP, the PADP may not reflect LVEDP. In patients with normal ventricular function, PADP correlates with LVEDP (27, 29). In patients with left ventricular dysfunction, a linear correlation may exist between the PADP and LVEDP, but LVEDP is typically greater than PADP (27, 29, 34, 35). Bouchard et al. (29) noted an increase in the disparity of PADP and LVEDP with pharmacologic interventions and with increasing heart rates. LVEDP decreased and PADP increased such that in 8 of 9 patients PADP was greater than 12 mm Hg with normal LVEDP. The pulmonary artery "a" wave correlated well with LVEDP (27) but can not consistently be determined (29, 35). As previously stated for PWP, PADP correlated well with the pre-a wave left ventricular pressure (29, 35, 66).

Despite these previous findings, Scheinman et al. (67) found a significant correlation between PAEDP and LVEDP in 25 patients in shock (12 with acute myocardial infarction). After the use of oxygen or inotropic agents, the PAEDP continued to correlate with LVEDP. Except for one patient, patients with PAEDP $>$ 15 mm Hg had LVEDP $>$ 12 mm Hg, and all patients with PAEDP $<$ 10 mm Hg had LVEDP $<$ 12 mm Hg. The better correlation in patients with shock was attributed to the fact that these patients do not have the changes in left ventricular compliance found in patients with chronic cardiac disorders, have a shift of ventricular function to a different point on a nonlinear pressure-volume curve, or have a diminished force of atrial contraction and/or a critical decrease in atrial stroke volume (67).

Despite the aforementioned correlations of pulmonary pressures with left ventricular pressures, it is important to note the instances in which these relationships do not pertain. The major disorders include pulmonary vascular disease, pulmonary venous or mitral obstruction, right bundle branch block, aortic insufficiency, and left atrial pressures below pulmonary capillary "critical closing" pressures (68).

Pulmonary artery pressures (PASP, PADP, and MPAP) are elevated in 1) states of increased pulmonary artery flow as in left to right shunts; 2) states of increased pulmonary vascular resistance secondary to cardiac dysfunction, pulmonary venous obstruction, or chronic lung disease; 3) hypoxia; 4) pulmonary emboli; 5) all causes of increased PWP; 6) too much or too rapid parenteral fluid administration. In general, caution must be used in interpreting a single pressure measurement. Sequential measurements are therefore essential. The frequency of measurements will obviously depend on the degree of hemodynamic instability in the individual patient. Recordings may be required as often as every 30 seconds or as infrequently as every hour. The hemodynamic alterations of the common cardiopulmonary disease states are shown in Table 4.2.

F. Mixed Venous Oxygen Tension

Mixed venous oxygen saturation (svO_2) is a useful index of effective systemic perfusion or tissue oxygenation because it is directly proportional to cardiac output when arterial oxygen content and tissue oxygen consumption remain constant. The arterial and mixed venous oxygen tensions (pvO_2) may be used to estimate the cardiac output (Fick method), oxygen consumption, and pulmonary shunt. In general, a decrease in cardiac output results in greater oxygen extraction by peripheral tissues, and therefore, abnormally low oxygen saturation is found in the venous blood returning to the heart. The normal mixed venous oxygen tension is 36-42 mm Hg. High pvO_2 may be seen in left to right shunts, septic shock, hyperbaric oxygenation, excess inotrope administration, and poor sampling technique. Low pvO_2 is found in patients with decreased cardiac output, hypoxemia, anemia, or high affinity hypoxia. Serum lactate levels increase as the venous oxygen tension falls below 27 mm Hg and unconsciousness occurs at levels of 18-20 mm Hg. Samples of mixed venous blood are unreliable in patients with left to right shunts and in some patients with severe mitral insufficiency because of retrograde flow associated with regurgitation.

Mixed venous blood samples are usually obtained from the pulmonary artery or right ventricle. Before the advent of the pulmonary artery catheter,

Table 4.2. Hemodynamic alterations in different cardiopulmonary disorders

Diagnosis	RAP (mm Hg)	PASP (mm Hg)	PADP (mm Hg)	PWP (mm Hg)
Primary pulmonary disorder	↑	↑↑	↑↑	N,↓
Cardiogenic pulmonary edema	↑	↑	↑	↑↑
Cardiogenic shock	↑	↑	↑	↑↑
Hypovolemic shock	↓	↓	↓	↓
Right ventricular infarction	↑↑	N,↓	N,↓	N,↓
Cardiac tamponade	↑	↑	↑	↑

RAP, Right atrial pressure, PASP, pulmonary artery systolic pressure; PADP, pulmonary artery diastolic pressure; PWP, pulmonary artery wedge pressure.

samples were obtained from CVP catheters. Goldman (69) noted that central venous oxygen saturation (cvO_2) obtained from the superior vena cava (SVC) correlated with myocardial function in patients with myocardial infarction. When cvO_2 was less than 60%, evidence of heart failure was present; when cvO_2 was less than 45%, both heart failure and shock were present. Many studies have noted significant differences between cvO_2 and svO_2 (70-73). The differences between cvO_2 and svO_2 are believed to be secondary to the inadequate mixing of SVC and inferior vena cava (IVC) blood. Under normal circumstances, IVC blood has a higher saturation than SVC blood due to the highly saturated renal venous effluent. In a study of severely ill cardiac patients, Scheinman et al. (71) reported that cvO_2 reflected svO_2 only in patients not in shock or heart failure. Studies of healthy ambulatory subjects showed that svO_2 was significantly higher than cvO_2 (70). Several reports in critically ill patients, however, demonstrated higher cvO_2 than svO_2 (71, 72, 74). A possible explanation for the differences in cvO_2 and svO_2 in healthy and seriously ill patients may be found in the study of Lee et al. (73). Lee noted that normal patients had a higher IVC oxygen saturation than SVC saturation and therefore had a higher svO_2 than cvO_2 (SVC oxygen saturation). On the other hand, patients in shock had a higher SVC oxygen saturation compared to the IVC saturation, most likely due to a redistribution of blood flow away from the renal and mesenteric bed toward the coronary and cerebral circulation. Therefore, these patients had a higher cvO_2 (SVC sample) than svO_2. In contrast to cvO_2 from the SVC, other studies have noted that saturations from the right atrium did correlate well with svO_2 (71, 73). Use of cvO_2 rather than svO_2 for calculation of pulmonary shunt or arterial-venous oxygen content difference can also lead to substantial errors (72, 74). Despite these differences in absolute values noted above, good correlations have been noted between changes in cvO_2 compared to changes in svO_2 (71). Other studies have not confirmed these correlations with change (73). Because of the aforementioned data, it seems appropriate to use pulmonary artery samples rather than CVP samples for pvO_2 and svO_2.

Before using pulmonary artery blood samples for pvO_2, one must be aware of the sources of error related to sampling techniques. An increase of oxygen tension in the pulmonary artery leading to a falsely high pvO_2 may occur secondary to retrograde flow and contamination with pulmonary capillary blood or diffusion of oxygen through the wall of small pulmonary arteries (24, 75, 76). The most common cause of sampling errors is distal migration or wedging of the pulmonary artery catheter tip. Gross contamination of mixed venous samples may be easily recognized in the presence of bright red blood and extremely high oxygen tension. Unfortunately, situations occur which are not so obvious. Shapiro et al. (75) identified contaminated mixed venous samples by comparing the CO_2 tensions in blood obtained from systemic ($paCO_2$) and pulmonary ($pvCO_2$) arteries. All contaminated samples had CO_2 tension differences ($pvCO_2$ - $paCO_2$) that were negative, whereas the vast majority of true mixed venous samples had CO_2 differences that were positive.

A sample of mixed venous blood from a normally positioned catheter can be contaminated with pulmonary capillary blood only if antegrade flow of pulmonary artery blood is exceeded by the rate of its withdrawal. The possibility of this occurrence is increased if the diameter of the pulmonary artery and its blood flow are reduced by such factors as a decrease in venous return or cardiac output, an increase in pulmonary vascular resistance, or by mechanical ventilation, especially with positive end-expiratory pressure (77). Breathing high concentrations of oxygen can magnify any capillary contamination that is present and can further increase the oxygen tension of pulmonary capillary blood.

The rate of withdrawal of blood from a pulmonary artery catheter has been shown to influence pvO_2 in some studies (24, 75) but has not affected pvO_2 in others (75, 76). The investigations that did not find differences in pvO_2 based on withdrawal rates included patients who breathed spontaneously and received low concentrations of inspired oxygen (75, 76). In contrast, the patients studied by Suter et al. (24) were critically ill and received controlled mechanical ventilation with pure oxygen. The pvO_2 showed a significant increase in samples obtained from the distal segment of the pulmonary artery compared to the proximal portion. Progressively higher pvO_2s were found at faster withdrawal rates. The rate of withdrawal did not alter pvO_2 when blood was taken from the first 5 cm of the pulmonary artery. These results may have been related to the absence of spontaneous breathing, oxygen administration, or cardiopulmonary alterations. The same conclusions were found in dogs under similar conditions (75).

Unfortunately, contaminated mixed venous samples have been demonstrated even in the presence of a good pulmonary artery tracing (75). It is also possible that too much negative pressure on a sampling syringe may cause the catheter to migrate distally during sampling when the pressure tracing is unavailable for monitoring (75).

Based on the available information, the following recommendations would seem appropriate for obtaining pvO_2:

1. Withdraw samples from the most proximal pulmonary artery location as is feasible.
2. Withdraw blood at very slow rates, especially in patients receiving mechanical ventilation, high concentrations of inspired oxygen and in patients with cardiopulmonary disorders (i.e., the majority of patients requiring pulmonary artery catheterization).
3. Ascertain that the catheter is in the proper position before and after each blood sample is taken.

II. CALCULATED VARIABLES

A. Body Surface Area

Hemodynamic parameters vary with the size of an individual. Therefore, it is easier to interpret values which have been "indexed" by body surface area (BSA). The body surface area is calculated from a height-weight nomogram.

B. Cardiac Index

Cardiac index (CI) is derived by dividing cardiac output by body surface area. Cardiac index is typically increased in septic shock, hyperthermia, and thyrotoxicosis. Cardiac index is decreased in hypovolemic states, congestive heart failure, and in patients with pulmonary emboli.

$$CI = \frac{CO}{BSA}$$

C. Stroke Volume

Stroke volume (SV) is the volume of blood pumped by the heart with each contraction. Stroke volume is derived by dividing the cardiac output by the heart rate. It is elevated in bradycardia, hypertension, and hypervolemia. It is decreased in cardiogenic and hypovolemic shock.

$$SV = \frac{CO}{HR}$$

D. Stroke Volume Index

The stroke volume index (SVI), or stroke index (SI), is calculated by dividing the stroke volume by the body surface area or by dividing the cardiac index by the heart rate.

$$SI = \frac{SV}{BSA} = \frac{CI}{HR}$$

E. Vascular Resistance

As blood flows through the vascular system, there is a resistance to flow. The origin of the relationship of these variables is found in electrical circuitry and defined by Ohm's Law.

$$\text{Resistance} = \frac{\text{Pressure}}{\text{Flow}}$$

1. Systemic or Peripheral Vascular Resistance Systemic or peripheral vascular resistance (SVR) measures the resistance in the systemic circulation. It is calculated by dividing the mean arterial pressure minus the central venous pressure by the cardiac output and multiplying by 79.9, a conversion factor for adjusting to the proper units ($\text{dyne}\cdot\text{sec}\cdot\text{cm}^{-5}$). Because this calculation does not correct for variations in size, some physicians have divided by cardiac index rather than cardiac output. Therefore, systemic vascular resistance index equals SVR multiplied by BSA, not divided by BSA. Despite the logic of correcting for BSA, this practice is not commonly followed.

Because changes in length of the vascular beds are uncommon after growth is completed, changes in vascular resistance usually reflect either altered blood viscosity or a change in the radius of the vascular circuit. The autonomic nervous system and local metabolic factors control SVR. It is important to appreciate that calculations of SVR based on mean pressure and flow of the entire systemic circulation may not accurately reflect regional differences in vascular resistance.

$$\text{SVR} = \frac{\text{MAP} - \text{CVP}}{\text{CO}} \times 79.9$$

In patients with shock, a cardiac output measurement and calculation of the systemic vascular resistance can have diagnostic importance. A hyperdynamic response with increased cardiac output and decreased systemic vascular resistance is typically seen in septic shock, whereas a hypodynamic response with decreased cardiac output and increased systemic vascular resistance is observed in hypovolemic, cardiogenic, and obstructive types of shock. Resistance may be increased because of arteriolar vasoconstriction or systemic hypertension. Resistance may be decreased in patients with cirrhosis, arteriovenous fistula, thyrotoxicosis, and anemia.

2. Pulmonary Vascular Resistance Pulmonary vascular resistance (PVR) measures the resistance in the pulmonary circulation. It is calculated by dividing the mean pulmonary artery pressure minus the pulmonary artery wedge pressure by the cardiac output (or cardiac index) and multiplying by 79.9.

$$\text{PVR} = \frac{\text{MPAP} - \text{PWP}}{\text{CO}} \times 79.9$$

This calculation is influenced by alterations in left atrial pressure and, therefore, will not always provide information solely related to the pulmonary vasculature. It may give an assessment of the presence and degree of pulmonary vascular disease. The pulmonary circulation is quite dynamic and may be influenced by mechanical (changes in flow, volume, pressure, edema), neural (autonomic nervous system), and biochemical (acidosis, oxygen tension, catecholamines, serotonin, histamine, and prostaglandins) alterations. Pulmonary vascular resistance is increased with pulmonary emboli, both cardiac and noncardiac pulmonary edema, and congenital or valvular heart disease.

F. Left Ventricular Stroke Work

Left ventricular stroke work (LVSW) is the external work of the left ventricle during each contraction. Left ventricular stroke work is derived as the product of the stroke index, the mean arterial pressure minus the pulmonary artery wedge pressure, and a conversion factor (0.0136). The LVSW is decreased in hypovolemic, cardiogenic, and septic shock. It is elevated in some types of hypertension and traumatic shock.

$$LVSW = SI \times (MAP - PWP) \times 0.0136$$

G. Right Ventricular Stroke Work

Right ventricular stroke work (RVSW) evaluates the right ventricular work as opposed to left ventricular work. RVSW is calculated as the product of the stroke index, the mean pulmonary artery pressure minus central venous pressure, and a conversion factor (0.0136). It is usually elevated in patients with pulmonary hypertension.

$$RVSW = SI \times (MPAP - CVP) \times 0.0136$$

H. Oxygen Content

Oxygen content is the product of the hemoglobin (Hgb) concentration, the percentage of saturation of hemoglobin with oxygen, and 1.36 (the amount of oxygen carried by each gram of fully saturated hemoglobin) plus the product of the oxygen solubility in blood (0.003) and the oxygen tension in blood (arterial or mixed venous blood samples or the alveolar oxygen tension for capillary oxygen content). Because the product of the arterial or mixed venous oxygen tension and the oxygen solubility is negligible, it is often not included. The oxygen saturation should be measured directly and not calculated from the normal oxyhemoglobin dissociation curve because factors such as pH, temperature, and 2,3-diphosphoglyceric acid (DPG) may affect it. Direct measurement of oxygen content may also be performed by the Van Slyke method or commercially available oxygen content analyzers.

$$CaO_2 = Hgb \times \text{Arterial } O_2 \text{ saturation} \times 1.36 + (pO_2 \times 0.003)$$

I. Arteriovenous Oxygen Content Difference

Arteriovenous oxygen content difference ($avDO_2$) is the difference between the arterial oxygen content (CaO_2) and the mixed venous oxygen content (CvO_2). As tissue extraction increases and mixed venous oxygen content decreases, arteriovenous oxygen content differences increase. This typically occurs in patients with decreased cardiac output. Patients with septic shock, shunting, low hemoglobin concentrations, or low P_{50} levels will have decreased arteriovenous oxygen content differences. Arteriovenous oxygen content differences may more simply be calculated as the product of 1.36, the hemoglobin concentration, and the difference between arterial and mixed venous oxygen saturations.

$$avDO_2 = CaO_2 - CvO_2$$

J. Oxygen Delivery

Oxygen transport, or *oxygen delivery* or *oxygen availability*, is a measure of the oxygen delivered to the peripheral tissues and is dependent on adequate oxygenation, hemoglobin concentration, and cardiac output. Oxygen delivery is calculated by multiplying cardiac output by arterial oxygen content. Oxygen delivery is therefore decreased in patients with decreased cardiac output, anemia, or hypoxemia.

Oxygen supply in the tissues depends on both the transport ability of the vascular system (expressed as oxygen transport, calculated above) and the diffusional transport processes (78). The extravascular process is by physical diffusion and is dependent on the pressure head of oxygen and the geometry of the microvasculature and the tissues.

Under clinical circumstances, the vascular component may be calculated, whereas the importance of diffusion is, unfortunately, unknown. If cells are directly adjacent to capillaries, the importance of the distance for diffusion is negligible and oxygenation is primarily dependent on vascular transport. Under these conditions, a very low capillary pO_2 would be possible without tissue hypoxia and the resultant anaerobic metabolism. On the other hand, if diffusion occurs across significant distances, oxygen supply to the tissues is extremely dependent on diffusion and high capillary pO_2 must be maintained.

Venous pO_2 which reflects the lowest measurable oxygen pressure in the vascular system is a sensitive indicator of the still lower value at the tissue or cellular level. In fact, the venous pO_2 has been found to reflect tissue pO_2 in many instances. In general, the diffusion distances in most tissues are not small and anaerobic metabolism may occur when venous pO_2 falls to 30 mm Hg. Independent of diffusion, vascular oxygen transport must obviously be maintained to keep up with the metabolic requirements and to sustain venous pO_2 at normal levels.

After prolonged periods of low pvO_2 secondary to hypoxia or low flow states, it is possible that capillary density will increase and thereby minimize diffusional transportation. In fact, it may be difficult at times to discern whether a low pvO_2 represents an acute or chronic problem. The importance of serial samples, therefore, can not be overemphasized.

Despite the fact that mixed venous pO_2 is a function of oxygen transport, the quantitative change in pvO_2 depends on the qualitative changes in the determinants of oxygen transport (CO, Hgb, and pO_2). Obviously, if cardiac output changes, pvO_2 changes inversely as defined by the Fick equation. If oxygen transport is changed by varying CaO_2, however, the effect on pvO_2 will depend on how the change in CaO_2 is effected. The same CaO_2 can be obtained with a normal Hgb and normal pO_2 or with an increased Hgb and decreased pO_2. For the same cardiac output the oxygen transport may be identical but the pvO_2 may be very different. In general, the response of pvO_2 to changes in cardiac output and hemoglobin concentrations is most sensitive to the lower levels of cardiac output and hemoglobin. In addition, these effects are additive. Therefore, increases in Hgb from anemic levels are especially effective in increasing pvO_2 if the cardiac output is low. On the other hand, Hgb or cardiac output changes in high cardiac output or polycythemic states will have little effect in increasing pvO_2. These three variables (CO, Hgb and pO_2) are, however, exceedingly important in altering pvO_2 and a decrease in pvO_2 certainly warrants their determination.

$$O_2 \text{ Delivery} = CO \times CaO_2 \times 10$$

K. Oxygen Consumption

Oxygen consumption, or oxygen uptake (VO_2), represents the amount of oxygen extracted by the peripheral tissues. Oxygen consumption is calculated as the product of the cardiac output and the arteriovenous oxygen content difference.

$$VO_2 = CO \times (CaO_2 - CvO_2) \times 10$$

Oxygen consumption may also be measured by collecting expired air. Oxygen consumption is increased in sepsis, thyrotoxicosis, and postoperative patients.

L. Oxygen Utilization Ratio

Oxygen utilization ratio, or oxygen extraction ratio, is the amount of delivered oxygen which is consumed or in other words, the rate of oxygen uptake (VO_2) normalized for (or divided by) the oxygen transport. The oxygen utilization ratio is calculated as the arteriovenous oxygen content difference divided by the arterial oxygen content. When the ratio is high, inadequate oxygen delivery is present and demand exceeds supply. A decreased ratio is related to an excessive cardiac output or anatomic or physiologic shunting. Some investigators have used the reciprocal of the O_2 utilization ratio (O_2 transport/VO_2) which has been called the coefficient of oxygen delivery (COD).

$$\text{Oxygen utilization ratio} = \frac{CaO_2 - CvO_2}{CaO_2}$$

M. Veno-arterial Admixture

Veno-arterial admixture, or Pulmonary Shunt (Qs/Qt), measures the fraction of total blood flow that is not oxygenated during its passage through the lungs. The equation for calculating the shunt is:

$$\frac{Qs}{Qt} = \frac{CcO_2 - CaO_2}{CcO2 - CvO_{-2}}$$

where Qs/Qt is the percentage of total cardiac output (Qt) shunted through the lungs and CcO_2, CaO_2, CvO_2 are the pulmonary capillary, arterial, and mixed venous oxygen contents, respectively. The CcO_2 is calculated with the assumption that the alveolar pO_2 and pulmonary capillary pO_2 are identical. A change in cardiac output usually causes a similar change in veno-arterial admixture. The resultant effect on arterial blood oxygen content depends on whether the alteration in pulmonary shunt predominates over the change in mixed venous blood oxygen content (79). If, for example, cardiac output decreases, pO_2 will decrease only if pvO_2 decreases more than the venous admixture. Because cardiac and pulmonary failure frequently occur simultaneously, measurements of pulmonary shunt as an index of pulmonary parenchymal damage assist in distinguishing pulmonary and cardiac components of the alveolar-arterial oxygen tension gradient.

REFERENCES

1. Hurst, J. W. 1978. The Heart. 4th Edition. McGraw Hill Book Co., New York.
2. Braunwald, E. 1980. Heart Disease: A textbook of Cardiovascular Medicine. W. B. Saunders Co., Philadelphia.
3. Grossman, W. 1980. Cardiac Catheterization and Angiography. 2nd Edition. Lea and Febiger, Philadelphia.
4. The Society of Critical Care Medicine. 1980. Critical Care: State of the Art, Vol 1, Fullerton, Calif.
5. Spodick, D. H. 1980. Physiologic and prognostic implications of invasive monitoring: Undetermined risk/benefit ratios in patients with heart disease (Editorial). Am. J. Cardiol. 46:173-175.
6. Patterson, S. W., and Starling, E. H. 1914. On the mechanical factors which determine the output of the ventricles. J. Physiol. 48:357-379.
7. Calvin, J. E., Driedger, A. A., and Sibbald, W. J. 1981. Does the pulmonary capillary wedge pressure predict left ventricular preload in critically ill patients? Crit. Care Med. 9:437-443.
8. Covell, J. W., Ross, J., Taylor, R., Sonnenblick, E. H., and Braunwald, E. 1967. Effects of increasing frequency of contraction on the force velocity relation of the left ventricle. Cardiovasc. Res. 1:2-8.
9. Sarin, C. L., Yalav, E., Clement, A. J., and Braimbridge, M. V. 1970. The necessity for measurement of left atrial pressure after cardiac surgery. Thorax 25:185-189.
10. Bell, H., Stubbs, D., and Pugh, D. 1971. Reliability of central venous pressure as an indicator of left atrial pressure: A study in patients with mitral valve disease. Chest 59:169-173.

11. Civetta, J. M., and Gabel, J. C. 1972. Flow directed-pulmonary artery catheterization in surgical patients: Indications and modifications of technic. Ann. Surg. 176:753-756.
12. Byrick, R. J., and Nobel, W. H. 1978. Influence of elevated pulmonary vascular resistance on the relationship between central venous pressure and pulmonary artery occluded pressure following cardiopulmonary bypass. Can. Anaesth. Soc. J. 25:106-112.
13. Del Guercio, L. R. M., and Cohn, J. D. 1976. Monitoring: Methods and significance. Surg. Clin. North Am. 56:977-994.
14. Mangano, D. T. 1980. Monitoring pulmonary arterial pressure in coronary-artery disease. Anesthesiology 53:364-370.
15. Forrester, J. S., Diamond, G., McHugh, T. J., and Swan, H. J. C. 1971. Filling pressures in the right and left sides of the heart in acute myocardial infarction. N. Engl. J. Med. 285:190-193.
16. Toussaint, G. P. M., Burgess, J. H., and Hampson, L. G. 1974. Central venous pressure and pulmonary wedge pressure in critical surgical illness. Arch. Surg. 109:265-269.
17. Civetta, J. M., Gabel, J. C., and Laver, M. B. 1971. Disparate ventricular function in surgical patients. Surg. Forum 22:136-139.
18. DeLaurentis, D. A., Hayes, M., Matsumoto, T., and Wolferth, C. C. 1973. Does central venous pressure accurately reflect hemodynamic and fluid volume patterns in the critical surgical patient? Am. J. Surg. 126:415-418.
19. Hellems, H. K., Haynes, F. W., Dexter, L., and Kinney, T. D. 1948. Pulmonary capillary pressure in animals estimated by venous and arterial catheterization. Am. J. Physiol. 155:98-105.
20. Lagerlof, H., and Werko, L. 1949. Studies on the circulation of blood in man. Scand. J. Clin. Lab. Invest. 1:147-161.
21. Batson, G. A., Chandrasekhar, K. P., Payas, Y., and Rickards, D. F. 1972. Measurement of pulmonary wedge pressure by the flow directed Swan-Ganz catheter. Cardiovasc. Res. 6:748-752.
22. Rapaport, E., and Dexter, L. 1953. Pulmonary "capillary" pressure. Methods Med. Res. 7:85-93.
23. Lappas, D., Lell, W. A., Gabel, J. C., Civetta, J. M., and Lowenstein, E. 1973. Indirect measurement of left-atrial pressure in surgical patients—pulmonary-capillary wedge and pulmonary-artery diastolic pressures compared with left-atrial pressure. Anesthesiology 38:394-397.
24. Suter, P. M., Lindauer, J. M., Fairley, H. B., and Schlobohm, R. M. 1975. Errors in data derived from pulmonary artery blood gas values. Crit. Care Med. 3:175-181.
25. Pace, N. L. 1977. A critique of flow-directed pulmonary arterial catheterization. Anesthesiology 47:455-465.
26. Brewster, H., and McIlroy, M. B. 1973. Blood gas tensions and pH of pulmonary "wedge" samples in patients with heart disease. J. Appl. Physiol. 34:413-416.
27. Falicov, R. E., and Resnekov, L. 1970. Relationship of the pulmonary artery end-diastolic pressure to the left ventricular end-diastolic and mean filling pressures in patients with and without left ventricular dysfunction. Circulation 42:65-73.
28. Jenkins, B. S., Bradley, R. D., and Branthwaite, M. A. 1970. Evaluation of pulmonary arterial end-diastolic pressure as an indirect estimate of left atrial mean pressure. Circulation 42:75-78.
29. Bouchard, R. J., Gault, J. H., and Ross, J. 1971. Evaluation of pulmonary arterial end-diastolic pressure as an estimate of left ventricular end-diastolic pres-

sure in patients with normal and abnormal left ventricular performance. Circulation 44:1072-1079.
30. Epps, R. G., and Adler, R. H. 1953. Left atrial and pulmonary capillary pressures in mitral stenosis. Brit. Heart J. 15:298-304.
31. Fitzpatrick, G. F., Hampson, L. G., and Burgess, J. H. 1972. Bedside determination of left atrial pressure. C. M. A. J. 106:1293-1298.
32. Walston, A., and Kendall, M. E. 1973. Comparison of pulmonary wedge and left atrial pressure in man. Am. Heart J. 86:159-164.
33. Sapru, R. P., Taylor, S. H., and Donald K. W. 1968. Comparison of the pulmonary wedge pressure with the left ventricular end-diastolic pressure in man. Clin. Sci. 34:125-140.
34. Rahimtoola, S. H., Loeb, H. S., Ehsani, A., Sinno, M. Z., Chuquimia, R., Lal, R., Rosen, K. M., and Gunnar, R. M. 1972. Relationship of pulmonary artery to left ventricular diastolic pressures in acute myocardial infarction. Circulation 46:283-290.
35. Fisher, M. L., DeFelice, C. E., and Parisi, A. F. 1975. Assessing left ventricular filling pressure with flow-directed (Swan-Ganz) catheters. Chest 68:542-547.
36. Hobelmann, C. F., Smith, D. E., Virgilio, R. W., Shapiro, A. R., and Peters, R. M. 1974. Left atrial and pulmonary artery wedge pressure difference with positive end-expiratory pressure. Surg. Forum. 25:232-234.
37. Lozman, J., Powers, S. R., Older, T., Dutton, R. E., Roy, R. J., English, M., Marco, D., and Eckert, C. 1974. Correlation of pulmonary wedge and left atrial pressures. Arch. Surg. 109:270-277.
38. Qvist, J., Pontoppidan, H., Wilson, R. S., Lowenstein, E., and Laver, M. B. 1975. Hemodynamic responses to mechanical ventilation with PEEP: The effect of hypervolemia. Anesthesiology 42:45-55.
39. Hobelmann, C. F., Smith, D. E., Virgilio, R. W., Shapiro, A. R., and Peters, R. M. 1975. Hemodynamic alterations with positive end-expiratory pressure: The contribution of the pulmonary vasculature. J. Trauma 15:951-959.
40. Downs, J. B., Douglas, M. E., Sanfelippo, P. M., Stanford, W., and Hodges, M. R. 1977. Ventilatory pattern, intrapleural pressure, and cardiac output. Anesth. Analg. 56:88-95.
41. Scharf, S. M., Caldini, P., and Ingram, R. H. 1977. Cardiovascular effects of increasing airway pressure in the dog. Am. J. Physiol. 232:H35-H43.
42. Zapol, W. M., and Snider, M. T. 1977. Pulmonary hypertension in severe acute respiratory failure. N. Engl. J. Med. 296:476-480.
43. Roy, R., Powers, S. R., Feustel, P. J., and Dutton, R. E. 1977. Pulmonary wedge catheterization during positive end-expiratory pressure ventilation in the dog. Anesthesiology 46:385-390.
44. Manny, J., Patten, M. T., Liebman, P. R., and Hechtman, H. B. 1978. The association of lung distention, PEEP and biventricular failure. Ann. Surg. 187:151-157.
45. Cassidy, S. S., Robertson, C. H., Pierce, A. K., and Johnson, R. L. 1978. Cardiovascular effects of positive end-expiratory pressures in dogs. J. Appl. Physiol. 44:743-750.
46. Jardin, F., Farcot, J. C., Boisante, L., Curien, N., Margairaz, A., and Bouedaris, J. P. 1981. Influence of positive end-expiratory pressure on left ventricular performance. N. Engl. J. Med. 304:387-392.
47. Kane, P. B., Askanazi, J., Neville, J. F., Mon, R. L., Hanson, E. L., and Webb, W. R. 1978. Artifacts in the measurement of pulmonary artery wedge pressure. Crit. Care Med. 6:36-38.

48. Davison, R., Parker, M., and Harrison, R. A. 1978. The validity of determinations of pulmonary wedge pressure during mechanical ventilation. Chest 73:352-355.
49. Calvin, J. E., Driedger, A. A., and Sibbald, W. J. 1981. Positive end-expiratory pressure (PEEP) does not depress left ventricular function in patients with pulmonary edema. Am. Rev. Respir. Dis. 124:121-128.
50. Neville, J. F., Askanazi, J., Mon, R. L., Kane, P. B., Hanson, E. L., and Webb, W. R. 1975. Determinants of pulmonary artery wedge pressure. Surg. Forum 26:206-208.
51. Tooker, J., Huseby, J., and Butler, J. 1978. The effect of Swan-Ganz catheter height on the wedge pressure-left atrial pressure relationship in edema during positive-pressure ventilation. Am. Rev. Respir. Dis. 117:721-725.
52. Todd, T. R. J., Baile, E. M., and Hogg, J. C. 1978. Pulmonary arterial wedge pressure in hemorrhagic shock. Am. Rev. Respir. Dis. 118:613-616.
53. Shasby, D. M., Dauber, I. M., Pfister, S., Anderson, J. T., Carson, S. B., Manart, F., and Hyers, T. M. 1981. Swan-Ganz catheter location and left atrial pressure determine the accuracy of the wedge pressure when positive end-expiratory pressure is used. Chest 80:666-670.
54. West, J. B., Dollery, C. T., and Naimark, A. 1964. Distribution of blood flow in isolated lung: Relation to vascular and alveolar pressures. J. Appl. Physiol. 19:713-724.
55. Cross, C. J., Cain, H. D., Deaton, W. J., Summerhill, S., and Stevens, P. M. 1978. Vertical relationships of the pulmonary artery catheter tip and transducer reference point in estimation of the left atrial pressure. Am. Rev. Respir. Dis. 177(Abstract):105.
56. Kronberg, G. M., Quan, S. F., Schlobohm, R. M., Lindauer, J. M., and Goodman, P. C. 1979. Anatomic locations of the tips of pulmonary-artery catheters in supine patients. Anesthesiology 51:467-469.
57. Orta, D. A., Eisen, S., Yergin, B. M., and Olsen, G. N. 1979. Segmental pulmonary angiography in the critically ill patients using a flow-directed catheter. Chest 76:269-273.
58. Rao, B. S., Cohn, K. E., Eldridge, F. L., and Hancock, E. W. 1968. Left ventricular failure secondary to chronic pulmonary disease. Am. J. Med. 45:229-241.
59. Lockhart, A., Tzareva, M., Nader, F., Leblanc, P., Schrijen, F., and Sadoul, P. 1969. Elevated pulmonary artery wedge pressure at rest and during exercise in chronic bronchitis: Fact or fancy. Clin. Sci. 37:503-517.
60. Rice, D. L., Awe, R. J., Gaasch, W. H., Alexander, J. K., and Jenkins, D. E. 1974. Wedge pressure measurement in obstructive pulmonary disease. Chest 66:628-632.
61. Gabriel, S. 1971. The difference between the pulmonary artery diastolic pressure and the pulmonary wedge pressure in chronic lung disease. Acta Med. Scand. 190:555-559.
62. Jonsson, B., and Sanai, S. 1969. The reliability of diastolic pressure measurement in the pulmonary artery as an index of mean left atrial pressure. Cardiologia 54:329-335.
63. Forsberg, S. A. 1971. Relations between pressure in pulmonary artery, left atrium and left ventricle with special reference to events at end diastole. Brit. Heart J. 33:494-499.
64. Subramanian, V. A., Hai, M. A., Sherman, M. M., and Berger, R. L. 1975. Filling pressures of the heart following open-heart surgery. Surg. Forum 26:236-237.
65. Humphrey, C. B., Oury, J. H., Virgilio, R. W., Gibbons, J. A., Folkerth, T. L.,

Shapiro, A. R., and Fosburg, R. G. 1976. An analysis of direct and indirect measurements of left atrial filling pressure. J. Thorac. Cardiovasc. Surg. 71:643-647.
66. Balcon, R., Bennett, E. D., and Sowton, G. E. 1972. Comparison of pulmonary artery diastolic and left ventricular end diastolic pressure in patients with ischaemic heart disease. Cardiovasc. Res. 6:172-175.
67. Scheinman, M., Evans, T. G., Weiss, A., and Rapaport, E. 1973. Relationship between pulmonary artery end-diastolic pressure and left ventricular filling pressure in patients in shock. Circulation 47:317-324.
68. Herbert, W. H. 1972. Limitations of pulmonary artery end-diastolic pressure. N.Y. State J. Med. 72:229-232.
69. Goldman, R. H., Klughaupt, M., Metcalf, T., Spivack, A. P., and Harrison, D. C. 1968. Measurement of central venous oxygen saturation in patients with myocardial infarction. Circulation 38:941-946.
70. Barratt-Boyes, B. G., and Wood, E. H. 1957. The oxygen saturation of blood in the venae cavae, right-heart chambers, and pulmonary vessels of healthy subjects. J. Lab. Clin. Med. 50:93-106.
71. Scheinman, M. M., Brown, M. A., and Rapaport, E. 1969. Critical assessment of use of central venous oxygen saturation as a mirror of mixed venous oxygen in severely ill cardiac patients. Circulation 40:165-172.
72. Horovitz, J. H., Carrico, C. J., and Shires, G. T. 1971. Venous sampling sites for pulmonary shunt determinations in the injured patient. J. Trauma 2:911-914.
73. Lee, J., Wright, F., Barber, R., and Stanley, L. 1972. Central venous oxygen saturation in shock: A study in man. Anesthesiology 36:472-478.
74. Dongre, S. S., McAslan, T. C., and Shin, B. 1977. Selection of the source of mixed venous blood samples in severely traumatized patients. Anesth. Analg. 56:527-532.
75. Shapiro, H. M., Smith, G., Pribble, A. H., Murray, J. A., and Cheney, F. W. 1974. Errors in sampling pulmonary arterial blood with a Swan-Ganz catheter. Anesthesiology 40:291-295.
76. Mihm, F., Feeley, T. W., Rosenthal, M., and Raffin, T. A. 1980. The lack of effect of variable blood withdrawal rates on the measurement of mixed venous oxygen saturation. Chest 78:452-455.
77. Douglas, M. E. 1980. So much, so little. (Editorial). Chest 78:418.
78. Tenney, S. M., and Mithoefer, J. C. 1982. The relationship of mixed venous oxygenation to oxygen transport: With special reference to adaptions to high altitude and pulmonary disease. Am. Rev. Respir. Dis. 125:474-479.
79. Cheney, F. W., and Colley, P. S. 1980. The effect of cardiac output on arterial blood oxygenation. Anesthesiology 52:496-503.

Chapter 5

Clinical Case Studies Utilizing the Pulmonary Artery Catheter

Charles L. Sprung, Bradley H. Ruben, Joseph M. Civetta, and Lawrence J. Jacobs

PATIENT 1: PNEUMONIA VERSUS CONGESTIVE HEART FAILURE/Charles L. Sprung

A 49-year-old man was admitted after complaining of weakness, anorexia, nausea, vomiting, diarrhea, and a cough that had lasted 2 weeks. The patient had a temperature of 103° F with shaking chills for the last 2 days. Well-differentiated, diffuse lymphocytic lymphoma was diagnosed 5 years before admission. Over the last few months the patient's course was complicated by paraplegia secondary to spinal cord compression by a tumor which partially resolved after radiotherapy. The patient had previously received chemotherapy with cyclophosphamide, vincristine, bleomycin, adriamycin, and prednisone.

Physical exam revealed a cachectic man in minimal distress. The temperature was 102.6° F; pulse, 110 beats/min; blood pressure (BP), 124/74 mm Hg; and respirations, 20 breaths/min. Generalized alopecia was noted. A 2 cm × 3 cm mass in the left posterior cervical area and bilateral matted inguinal lymph nodes were palpated. The chest was clear to percussion and auscultation, and the heart exam was without murmurs or gallops. There was mild tenderness in the lower abdomen, but no hepatosplenomegaly; bowel sounds were normal. Bilateral costovertebral angle (CVA) tenderness was present. An old, healing sacral decubitus (10 cm) without tenderness, erythema, warmth, or exudate was also noted. Neurologic examination demonstrated an oriented man with previously present muscle weakness in the lower extremities.

Laboratory data included a chest x-ray with a previously noted right hilar mass and a normal electrocardiogram (ECG). White blood cell count was 29,000/cu mm with a shift to the left, hematocrit (Hct) 21%; and platelets, 68,000/cu mm. The blood urea nitrogen (BUN) was 23 mg/dl; creatinine, 1.4 mg/dl; total protein, 5.1 grams/dl; and albumin, 2.9 grams/dl. Urinalysis revealed white blood cells that were too numerous to count and 4+ bacteria. The patient was treated for urosepsis with cephalothin and tobramycin and was transfused. The urine and blood cultures subsequently grew *Staphylococcus aureus.* After 2 days, the peripheral white blood cell count returned to normal and the patient became afebrile. Subsequently, the patient continued to have shaking chills with temperature elevations to 102° F despite antibiotic therapy. A right lower lobe pneumonia was found. Sputum grams stains and cultures were not helpful and erythromycin was started to cover an atypical pneumonia which was felt to be unlikely but worth treating. During the hospitalization, the patient's serum protein concentration decreased further, despite hyperalimentation, and he developed anasarca. The patient developed dyspnea and rales were heard over the entire right side and half the way up the left side of the chest. The patient was also hypoxic at this time and required an inspired oxygen concentration (FIO_2) of 40% to maintain an arterial oxygen tension (pO_2) above 60 mm Hg. The repeat chest x-ray can be seen in Figure 5.1. Because of the inability to determine by clinical means whether the diffuse bilateral pulmonary infiltrates were secondary to congestive heart failure (no S_3 gallop was heard), volume overload secondary to a low protein and colloid osmotic pressure (1), or progressive pneumonia, a pulmonary artery catheter was inserted. The cardiac output was 9.0 liters/min; cardiac index; 4.4 liters/min/m^2; central venous pressure (CVP), 2 mm Hg; pulmonary artery pressure, 35/12 mm Hg; and pulmonary artery wedge pressure (PWP); 5 mm Hg. The colloid osmotic pressure was 14.7 mm Hg. Because of the progressive pneumonia in an immunocompromised host, an open lung biopsy was performed.

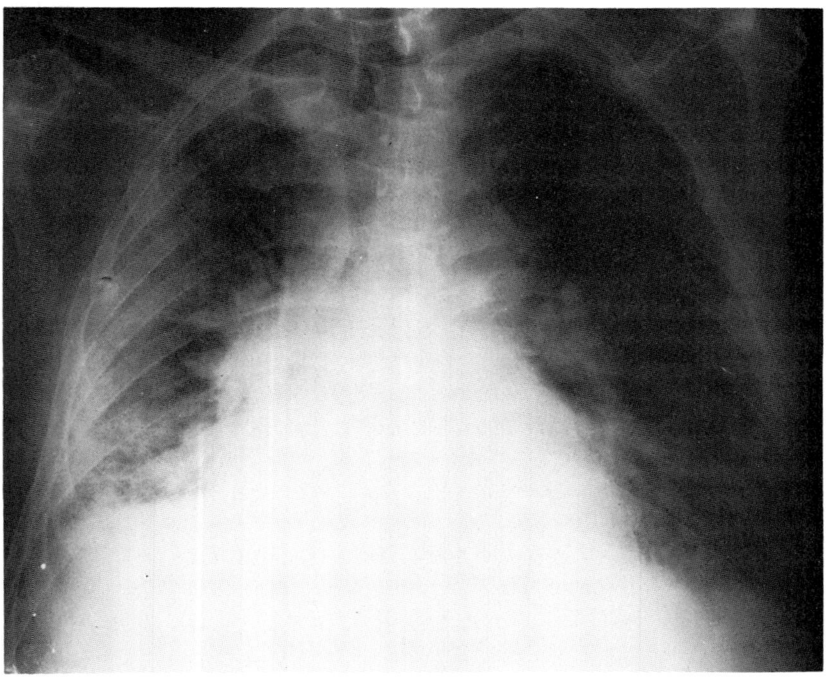

Figure 5.1. Pulmonary roentgenogram demonstrating diffuse bilateral infiltrates. Pulmonary artery catheterization was performed to differentiate between pneumonia or congestive heart failure as an etiology.

Discussion

Pulmonary artery catheterization has become an essential tool in differentiating cardiac from pulmonary etiologies of respiratory distress and bilateral pulmonary infiltrates. The original pulmonary artery catheter did not have the capability of performing cardiac output determinations. The catheter's major utility was to measure hydrostatic pressures, especially the pulmonary artery wedge pressure which reflects left atrial pressure. By measuring these pressures, the cardiac and pulmonary contributions to the patient's problem could be more accurately defined. The addition of cardiac output measurements can be of further help. The patient with congestive heart failure has a decreased cardiac output and an increased PWP and CVP, whereas the patient with a pulmonary disorder has a normal or increased cardiac output, a normal or low PWP, and a CVP that may be elevated. In addition, the gradient between the pulmonary artery diastolic pressure and the PWP is usually normal in patients with cardiac disorders, but increased in primary pulmonary abnormalities. The patient with volume overload has an elevated PWP and CVP, despite a normal cardiac output.

Many patients who are presently being admitted to intensive care units have multiple organ failure. Because of the complexity of their disease, it may be extremely difficult by clinical means to identify the respiratory and cardiac contributions to their disease. The present patient is a good example, as he had several medical problems. The etiology of his respiratory failure was not certain, although the clinical suspicion was that it was infectious. Possible etiologies for the pulmonary disease included 1) a bacterial (previous *staph* infection), fungal (yeast had been seen and cultured in the urine), viral, tuberculous, or atypical pneumonia; 2) the patient's previous chemotherapy (bleomycin or cyclophosphamide) (2) or radiation to the chest; 3) volume overload; and 4) congestive heart failure. If volume overload or congestive heart failure was present and could be effectively treated, it was felt an open lung biopsy might be avoided. The elevated cardiac output and index and consistently low or normal PWP effectively ruled out congestive heart failure or volume overload. The pulmonary artery catheter, therefore, helped to exclude these as etiologies of the respiratory disorder. In view of the ineffective treatment of this unknown process in this immunocompromised patient, an open lung biopsy was performed. Pathologic examination revealed an interstitial pneumonitis. Stains for bacteria, acid fast bacillus (AFB), and fungus were negative. Lung tissue sent to the Centers for Disease Control (CDC) was positive for *Legionella dunofii*. The erythromycin which was started because of its minimal toxicity but without a strong clinical indication was probably lifesaving. The patient was discharged from the intensive care unit (ICU) and within a few days became afebrile.

PATIENT 2: COMPLICATED MYOCARDIAL INFARCTION/ Charles L. Sprung

A 66-year-old man with a history of previous myocardial infarction, congestive heart failure and ventricular arrhythmias was admitted complaining of several hours of dull substernal chest pain. The pain did not radiate and was associated with diaphoresis and a feeling of impending syncope. Three sublingual nitroglycerin tablets did not relieve the pain. The patient's previous medication included digoxin, furosemide, quinidine sulfate, and potassium chloride.

Physical examination revealed: blood pressure, 100/70 mm Hg; pulse, 96 beats/min; respirations, 18 breaths/min; bilateral basilar rales, point of maximal impulse (PMI) at the 6th intercostal space, 2 cm lateral to the midclavicular line; and an S_4 gallop.

Laboratory data showed a white blood count of 12,000/cu mm; hematocrit, 42.9%; and an arterial blood gas (2 liters oxygen by nasal cannula), pH 7.48; pO_2, 81 mm Hg; and arterial carbon dioxide tension (pCO_2), 30 mm Hg. Chest roentgenogram demonstrated cardiomegaly and evidence of vascular redistribution. The admission electrocardiogram revealed an acute inferior myocardial infarction.

Hospital Course

The patient's continued chest pain was relieved by 5 mg of morphine sulfate. Frequent multifocal premature ventricular contractions including couplets were treated with a bolus and continuous drip of lidocaine hydrochloride. Cardiac enzymes were positive with a creatine phosphokinase (CPK) of 1065 international units (IU) and positive MB bands.

Several episodes of junctional rhythms with ventricular rates of 40-50 beats/ min were associated with hypotension (BP, 70/50 mm Hg). The bradycardia responded to atropine, and a temporary transvenous pacemaker was inserted. Several hours later the patient again became hypotensive (BP, 75/50 mm Hg) despite a ventricular response of 70 beats/min. The patient was given a fluid challenge of 100 ml of normal saline over 10 minutes without an increase in blood pressure. A dopamine drip was started and pulmonary artery catheterization was performed. The results of the first hemodynamic profile can be seen in Profile Chart 5.1 (Profile #1).

Nitroprusside was added to the dopamine and a repeat hemodynamic profile was performed (Profile Chart 5.1, profile #2). In an attempt to increase the cardiac output the pacemaker rate was increased (Profile Chart 5.1, profile #3).

Over the next few days, the PWP was kept as high as possible to maximize cardiac output but to avoid pulmonary edema. Normal sinus rhythm returned and the patient was weaned from the dopamine and nitroprusside successfully.

Profile Chart 5.1 Cardiopulmonary profile of patient with a complicated myocardial infarction

Enter:	Date/time:	# 1	# 2	# 3
Cardiac output (CO)		3.2	3.6	3.9
Systolic blood pressure (SBP)		100	100	105
Diastolic blood pressure (DBP)		70	62	72
Mean arterial pressure (MAP)		80	75	83

Profile Chart 5.1. (Continued)

Heart rate (HR)	70	65	102
Mean pulmonary artery pressure (MPAP)	32	26	28
Pulmonary artery wedge pressure (PWP)	27	21	20
Central venous pressure (CVP)	25	18	16
Body surface area (BSA)	1.5	1.5	1.5
Data:			
Stroke volume (SV)	45.7	55.4	38.2
Cardiac index (CI)	2.1	2.4	2.6
Stroke index (SI)	30.5	36.9	25.5
Right ventricular stroke work (RVSW)	3	4	4
RVSW/CVP ratio	0.12	0.22	0.25
Left ventricular stroke work (LVSW)	22	27	22
LVSW/PWP ratio	0.81	1.29	1.1
Systemic vascular resistance (SVR)	1373	1265	1373
Pulmonary vascular resistance (PVR)	125	111	164
Enter:			
Hemoglobin (Hgb)	13.2	13.2	13.2
FIO_2	0.4	0.4	0.4
$PaCO_2$	34	36	37
PaO_2	69	74	85
SaO_2	0.94	0.95	0.96
PvO_2	27	30	32
SvO_2	0.52	0.60	0.63
DATA:			
Capillary O_2 content (CcO_2)	18.7	18.7	18.7
Mixed Venous O_2 content (CvO_2)	9.4	10.9	11.4
Arterial O_2 content (CaO_2)	17.1	17.3	17.5
Arteriovenous O_2 content difference ($avDO_2$)	7.7	6.4	6.1
O_2 delivery	547	623	683
O_2 consumption (VO_2)	246	230	238
O_2 utilization ratio	0.45	0.37	0.35
Intrapulmonary shunt (Qs/Qt)	0.17	0.18	0.16
PaO_2/FIO_2	173	185	213

Vasopressors or vasodilators (μ/k/m)	Dopa 5	Dopa 5/	Dopa 5/
PEEP		Nipride 1	Nipride 1
Respirator rate			
Tidal volume			
PIP			

Discussion

Experience in the coronary care unit and extensive research on acute myocardial infarction during the past decade have substantially altered the management of this serious disorder. In-hospital mortality has decreased from 30% to 15% with the advent of coronary care units and the availability of treatment for arrhythmias. Attention is now focused on the other major complication of acute myocardial infarction, mechanical "pump failure," and the hope of salvaging ischemic myocardium. Pump failure remains the major cause of hospital mortality in patients with myocardial infarction. There is a wide range of ventricular function in patients with acute myocardial infarction. One-third of patients will have normal left ventricular function during the period of their acute infarction. The extent of infarction is often correlated with the presence and degree of pump failure. In addition, the level of left ventricular function has a direct relation to hospital mortality. Therefore, it is not surprising that clinical or hemodynamic classifications are good indices of survival.

The Killip clinical classification separates patients into four groups (3):

Class I, No signs of pulmonary congestion
Class II, Moderate heart failure evidenced by tachypnea, rales at the lung bases and an S_3 gallop
Class III, Severe heart failure
Class IV, Shock

The mortalities for the four classes are 0-5%, 10-20%, 35-45%, and 85-95%, respectively. Forrester et al. (4) have compared a clinical classification based on pulmonary congestion and peripheral hypoperfusion with a hemodynamic classification. The clinical classification is:

Class I, No pulmonary congestion or peripheral hypoperfusion
Class II, Pulmonary congestion without hypoperfusion
Class III, Peripheral hypoperfusion without congestion
Class IV, Both hypoperfusion and congestion

The hemodynamic correlate of this classification based on the pulmonary artery wedge pressure (greater than or less than or equal to 18 mm Hg) and the cardiac index (greater than or less than or equal to 2.2 liters/min/m^2) can be seen in Table 5.1. The clinical classification correctly predicts the hemodynamic subset in approximately 70% of patients. It is therefore not surprising that the mortality rates of both the clinical and hemodynamic classifications are comparable. Clinical criteria are a valid reflection of cardiac hemodynamics in the majority of patients. Unfortunately, clinical prediction of the hemodynamic state may be incorrect in 15% of patients with PWP greater than 18 mm Hg and 25% of patients with cardiac indices less

Table 5.1. Mortality rates in clinical and hemodynamic subsets

Subset	Pulmonary congestion[a]	Peripheral hypoperfusion[b]	% Mortality	
			Clinical	Hemodynamic
I	-	-	1	3
II	+	-	11	9
III	-	+	18	23
IV	+	+	60	51

[a]Pulmonary-capillary pressure > 18 mm Hg
[b]Cardiac index < 2.2 liters/min/m²

than 2.2 liter/min/m². The latter error typically occurs in patients with pulmonary congestion. The importance of recognizing peripheral hypoperfusion is underscored by the markedly increased mortality in its presence (Figure 5.2).

Pulmonary artery catheterization during acute myocardial infarction is performed for the following indications which are more fully discussed in Chapter 1. These include: hypotension, congestive heart failure, sinus tachycardia, hypertension, acute mitral regurgitation, ventricular septal defect, pericardial tamponade, right ventricular infarction, and the assessment of interventions to decrease myocardial infarct size.

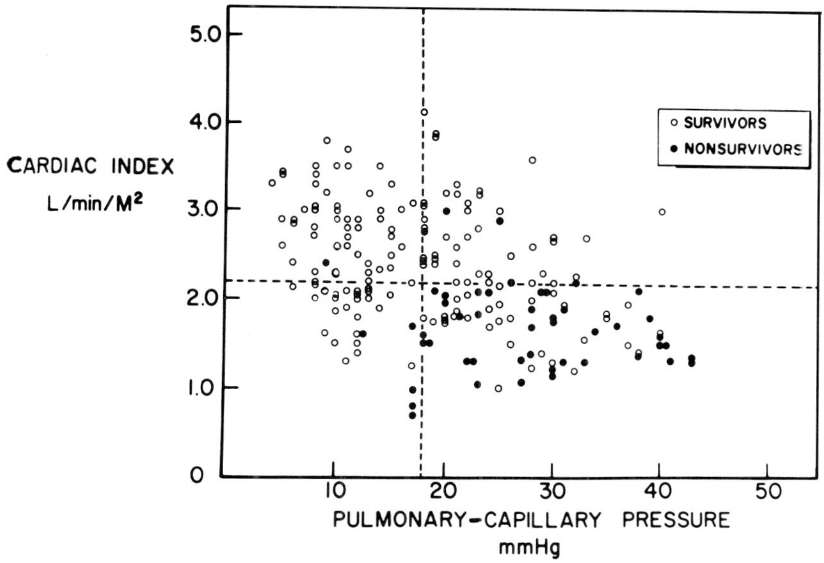

Figure 5.2. The relation between pulmonary artery wedge pressure (PWP) and cardiac index in patients admitted with acute myocardial infarction. The dotted lines are at PWP levels of 18 mm Hg and cardiac indices of 2.2 liters/min/m². Note that there is a wide range of left ventricular performance in patients with acute myocardial infarction and that mortality increases as cardiac performance deteriorates. Reproduced from Forrester et al., 1976 (4) with permission.

Assuming pulmonary artery catheterization was performed for one of the above indications, hemodynamic evaluation will place the patient in one of the four hemodynamic subsets. Based on this information, pulmonary congestion is relieved by decreasing elevated PWP and hypoperfusion is improved by increasing low cardiac output. It is the physician's hope that by performing these maneuvers, ischemic myocardium will not undergo infarction and the patient's chance for survival will improve. These ends are probably realized if the imbalance between myocardial oxygen supply and demand is not affected adversely by therapy. The amount of oxygen delivered to the myocardium is the product of coronary blood flow and arterial oxygen content. As opposed to other tissues which can increase oxygen extraction dependent on needs, normal myocardial tissue has near maximal extraction rates even under conditions of rest. An increase in oxygen demand is met by an increase in coronary flow. Unfortunately, a patient with a fixed coronary lesion may not be able to increase flow and may develop further ischemia or infarction. Under these circumstances, medical therapy offers little to increase oxygen supply but may be of substantial benefit in decreasing myocardial oxygen demands. Decreasing an elevated PWP may, however, increase coronary perfusion. Because there is a variable response to therapy in each of the hemodynamic subsets, the choice of therapy for a specific patient will be determined by the level of PWP and cardiac output. Therefore, the criteria for therapy of altered cardiac function are based on the assessment of the hemodynamic data in a given patient and knowledge of the effect of the therapeutic modality on both cardiac functions and metabolism.

The following is a discussion of the therapeutic modalities available in each of the subsets as described by Forrester et al. (4).

The uncomplicated patient (subset I) usually has normal hemodynamic parameters and therapy is not generally required. Many of these patients will have evidence of systolic hypertension, tachycardia, or even increased pulmonary artery wedge pressures. Many of these patients respond to bed rest and sedation. Despite the theoretical benefits of correcting these determinants of myocardial oxygen consumption, there are no data in man to recommend the use of propranolol (for tachycardia and hypertension), antihypertensives, oxygen, steroids, glucose-insulin-potassium or other modalities. Recently, however, beta-blocking agents have been shown to decrease mortality after myocardial infarction (5).

The patient with pulmonary congestion and no peripheral hypoperfusion is classified as subset II. Therapy is aimed at decreasing the PWP below the level causing pulmonary congestion but above the level which would cause a decrease in cardiac output by the Starling mechanism. In patients with myocardial infarction this can usually be accomplished by decreasing the PWP to 15-18 mm Hg. At this level, pulmonary congestion will disappear after 12-48 hours (6) and there is minimal or no decrease in cardiac output (7). This can be accomplished because of the exponential shape of the ventricular pressure-volume curve and the logarithmic shape of the Starling curve as shown in Figure 5.3. When PWP is high, a small change in ventricular volume causes a large decrease in PWP. This small decrease in volume, however, causes very little decrease in cardiac output. Thereafter, a further reduction in PWP can cause large reductions in volume and cardiac output. Therefore, if PWP is decreased to 0-10 mm Hg, substantial decreases in cardiac output can occur. The PWP can be measured serially with the cardiac output and a Starling curve can be constructed for the individual patient. Thus, an optimal PWP with maximum cardiac output can be obtained for that patient.

A decrease in PWP can be accomplished by diuretics, vasodilators, or inotropic agents. Furosemide is typically used as a diuretic. It increases venous capacitance even before its diuretic effect (8). Furosemide (20 mg) offers a wide margin of safety (vasodilators are more potent and are continuously administered intravenously) and do not increase myocardial oxygen demand (as the inotropes). The two most commonly used vasodilators are nitroglycerin and nitroprusside. Nitroglycerin predominantly dilates the venous system, whereas nitroprusside is both an arterial and venous vasodilator. Therefore, nitroglycerin may be appropriate for the patient with pulmonary congestion and continued chest pain, whereas nitroprusside may be

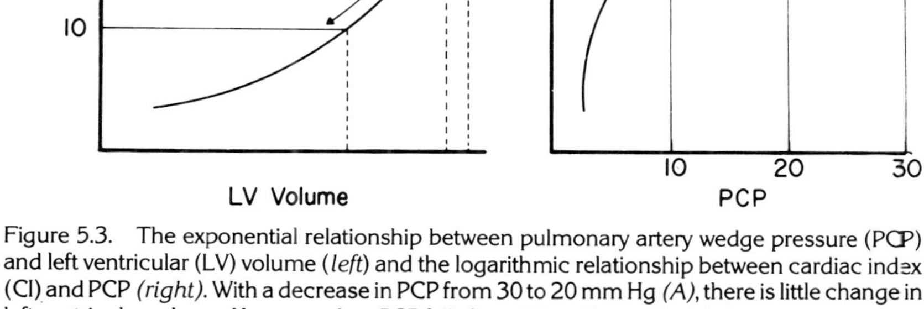

Figure 5.3. The exponential relationship between pulmonary artery wedge pressure (PCP) and left ventricular (LV) volume (*left*) and the logarithmic relationship between cardiac index (CI) and PCP *(right)*. With a decrease in PCP from 30 to 20 mm Hg *(A)*, there is little change in left ventricular volume. However when PCP falls from 20 to 10 mm Hg (*B*), there is a substantial decrease in left ventricular volume. The different responses in cardiac index to these same reductions in PCP can be seen on the right. With a small change in left ventricular diastolic volume (*A*), there is little change in preload and little change in cardiac output. When preload is substantially reduced by a reduction in PCP (*B*), however, a significant reduction in cardiac output may occur. Reproduced from Forrester et al., 1976 (4) with permission.

more applicable to the patient with congestion and systemic hypertension. If one decreases the increased systemic arterial pressure and PWP, it is probable that myocardial oxygen demands will also decrease. However, it is also possible that a reduction in aortic diastolic pressure might result in a decrease in myocardial oxygen supply.

Inotropes such as digitalis, dopamine, or dobutamine can also be used in patients with acute myocardial infarction and congestive heart failure. The use of digitalis in the face of an acute infarction remains controversial (9). Because of the potential for increased myocardial oxygen demand with an inotrope, we have tended to avoid the inotropic agents, if possible. These patients can usually be treated with diuretics or vasodilators and may not require inotropes.

Some patients who appear to have pulmonary congestion clinically have been shown to have normal PWP (10). This is especially true of the patient who has recently been treated for congestive heart failure. A rapid decrease in PWP to the normal range can be accompanied by a "lag phase" and persistence of rales and roentgenographic evidence of congestion (6). A further decrease in PWP with a diuretic or vasodilator could decrease the cardiac output dramatically and prove disastrous.

Peripheral hypoperfusion without pulmonary congestion (subset III) is usually treated by increasing cardiac output. The methods employed include volume expansion, increasing heart rate, and inotropes. Volume infusions are typically used in patients with low or normal PWP. By increasing PWP, the cardiac output increases by the Starling mechanism (see Figure 5.3). Unfortunately the Starling curve is rarely normal in patients with acute myocardial infarction and the increase in cardiac output may not be great. There is usually little increase in cardiac output beyond a PWP of 15-18 mm Hg (7), but increases can occasionally be seen at PWP of 20-25 mm Hg. It is therefore important to construct a curve for each patient and determine the optimal PWP. Some patients in this subset have a decreased cardiac output on the basis of an inappropriately low heart rate. The stroke volume in these patients may be normal. An increase in heart rate may be helpful in increasing cardiac output and peripheral perfusion. This typically occurs in patients with pulse rates of 50-70 beats/min. Atropine is usually not recommended because it may cause excessive tachycardia and/or increase the risk of arrhythmias. Therefore, temporary transvenous pacemakers may afford a safer alternative, despite the added invasive procedure. Finally, vasopressors may be required to maintain perfusion if volume infusions and/or pacing are inadequate. The usual sequence of treatment is volume resuscitation or pacemaker insertion followed by vasopressors. It is believed that this sequence yields the greatest benefits and least risks to the patient with an acute infarction. It should be recognized that all of these therapeutic modalities may increase myocardial ischemia by increasing myocardial oxygen demand (by increasing heart size, heart rate, or contractility).

The mortality of infarction increases dramatically in the patient with both peripheral hypoperfusion and pulmonary congestion (subset IV). Most patients in the previous subset who do not respond to therapy, rapidly join this subset with its poor prognosis. The goal of therapy in this group is to improve cardiac output, and at the same time, to decrease PWP. Obviously, hemodynamic monitoring is the preferred method used to treat such patients. If systemic vascular resistance (SVR) is increased, vasodilators such as nitroprusside (which affect preload and afterload) may be used. Typically, a decrease in SVR and PWP is accompanied by an increase in cardiac output and a minimal decrease or no change in blood pressure and pulse. These changes should dictate a reduction in myocardial oxygen demand. However, nitroprusside may increase dp/dt (an indicator of myocardial oxygen demand) and coronary perfusion pressure may also decrease. These agents must be used with extreme caution if a patient's blood pressure is low.

Vasopressors or inotropes (such as dopamine, dobutamine, and norepinephrine) may also be required. These agents are typically used when systolic pressures are below 90-100 mm Hg. They increase myocardial contractility and may increase aortic diastolic pressure, coronary perfusion, and myocardial oxygen supply with their increase in blood pressure. Unfortunately, oxygen demands are typically increased by vasopressor agents. Vasopressors are typically titrated to maintain an optimal level of arterial pressure. This level is determined by the patient's clinical response (increased urine output, improved mental status, and decreased arteriovenous oxygen content difference ($avDO_2$) and lactate concentration) and usually corresponds to a systolic pressure of 90-110 mm Hg. Unfortunately, inotropic agents are less effective in patients with large infarctions and severe left ventricular failure. Ironically, those patients who require inotropes most show the least response to these agents. In addition to the use of vasodilators and vasopressors alone, these agents can be used in combination (11). Dopamine may be used to increase the blood pressure above 100 mm Hg and nitroprusside may then be added for vasodilation. Dopamine can then be increased for any decrease in blood pressure with nitroprusside therapy. Finally, a marked improvement in cardiac output may be accomplished with the use of the intra-aortic balloon pump. The balloon is deflated at the onset of systole. This decreases the resistance to ejection and aortic diastolic pressure and coronary perfusion pressure increase. These changes undoubtedly decrease myocardial oxygen demands. This procedure may be so effective as to reverse cardiogenic shock. Unfortunately this is only a short-term method to maintain perfusion. The initial etiology of hypoperfusion (myocardial infarction and/or ischemia) must be effectively treated for the mechanical assistance to be beneficial on a long-term basis.

Despite the sound theoretical basis for the above physiologic approach to therapeutics as first espoused by Forrester et al. (4) and the use of these principles for the care of patients throughout the world, there are no data to indicate that these therapies decrease infarct size or improve long-term survival in man. Until these data become available, however, this physiologic approach based on clinical and hemodynamic information appears appropriate.

The present patient was initially hypotensive secondary to bradycardia which responded quite well to atropine. Because of the high degree of atrioventricular block and bradycardia, a prophylactic pacemaker was inserted. When hypotension recurred with a normal sinus rhythm, incipient cardiogenic shock was suspected and a fluid infusion was begun. It became clear quite quickly that volume would not reverse the hypotension in this patient. Therefore, dopamine was started to maintain adequate perfusion and pulmonary artery catheterization was performed. The initial hemodynamic profile (see Profile Chart 5.1, profile #1) revealed both hypoperfusion and congestion, which were evident clinically. The decreased cardiac index, stroke index, left ventricular stroke work (LVSW), and elevated PWP and SVR denoted a patient in subset IV. The pulse was only 70 beats/min despite the shock state, presumably because of the underlying conduction system disease. Despite an adequate hemoglobin and arterial oxygen saturation, the depressed myocardial function led to a very low oxygen delivery and a markedly increased $avDO_2$ and O_2 utilization ratio. These parameters of tissue perfusion were markedly abnormal, despite the normal pressure maintained by dopamine. The markedly increased CVP, which was almost equal to the PWP, may have been indicative of a right ventricular infarction. This patient had hypotension despite an elevated CVP and PWP, indicating significant left ventricular damage.

Because of the poor cardiac function and abnormal parameters of tissue perfusion, vasodilation was attempted. Vasodilation in the face of hypotension is difficult if not impossible. The use of dopamine to maintain adequate pressure allowed the addition of a vasodilator, nitroprusside. Repeat hemodynamics (profile #2) revealed an increase in CI, SI, and LVSW and a decrease in PWP, SVR, and $avDO_2$, and O_2 utilization ratio. Dobutamine could have been used as an inotrope instead of dopamine. Dobutamine can be especially useful in patients who have an increased PWP, as it tends to decrease PWP, whereas dopamine may increase PWP further by venoconstriction.

Finally, one must always remember that cardiac output can be increased by increasing heart rate. In patients with conduction disorders, ventricular pacing can increase cardiac output and allow the weaning of vasopressor agents. Unfortunately, ventricular pacing (profile #3) improved the patient only minimally if at all. This lack of substantial improvement may have been secondary to the loss of atrial kick that was previously present.

PATIENT 3: MITRAL REGURGITATION VERSUS VENTRICULAR SEPTAL DEFECT/Lawrence J. Jacobs

A 78-year-old man sought medical attention after experiencing recurrent substernal discomfort over a day. His electrocardiogram demonstrated an acute anterior wall myocardial infarction and he was admitted to the coronary care unit. His history was remarkable for "mild" hypertension and for the absence of clinical atherosclerotic or valvular heart disease. Physical examination on admission demonstrated a BP of 120/80 mm Hg; pulse, 90 beats/min; and regular and unlabored respirations. All peripheral pulses were palpated and were of normal quality; the neck veins were flat and the lungs clear. Cardiac exam revealed distant heart sounds; no murmurs, gallops, or rubs were auscultated. The remainder of the examination was unremarkable. Normal cardiac silhouette and clear lung fields were demonstrated on chest roentgenogram. Serial cardiac enzymes and isoenzymes ultimately confirmed the presence of myocardial necrosis with a peak CPK of 2,975 IU.

His initial course was uncomplicated by arrhythmias, congestive heart failure, or hypotension, and he was transferred from the coronary care unit on the fourth hospital day.

The subsequent 4 days were characterized by uneventful convalescence. On the ninth hospital day he complained of weakness. Physical examination revealed a new grade III/VI holosystolic murmur at the lower left sternal border, radiating to the axilla. On the following day the pulse rate was 100 beats/min and blood pressure 98/80 mm Hg. In addition to the murmur, a summation gallop was now heard. The chest roentgenogram showed new vascular fullness. The patient was transferred back to the coronary care unit.

To ascertain the nature of the new systolic murmur and the extent of hemodynamic compromise, a pulmonary artery catheter was inserted into the right pulmonary artery via the left subclavian vein. The following data were obtained:

	Oxygen saturation (%)	Pressure (mm Hg)
Inferior vena cava	64	
Right atrium	61	11 (mean)
Right ventricle	89	57/8
Right pulmonary artery	85	54/22
Pulmonary capillary wedge		24 (mean)
		V = 46
Radial artery	96	

The shunt was 3:1 and the hemoglobin was 12 grams/dl. Large V waves seen in the pulmonary capillary wedge pressure tracing indicated a high likelihood for the presence of mitral regurgitation (Figure 5.4). In addition, the significant step-up of oxygen saturation between the right atrium and right ventricle demonstrated the concomitant existence of a left to right shunt, reflecting acute rupture of the interventricular septum.

Although pulmonary flow determined by the thermodilution method usually equals systemic flow (cardiac output), the presence of a left to right shunt invalidates this equation. To determine systemic cardiac output it is necessary to calculate the pulmonary: systemic flow ratio. This is done by utilizing the formula for oxygen consumption:

$$O_2 \text{ consumption } (VO_2) = CO \times avDO_2$$

In the case of the present patient whose hemoglobin was 12 grams/dl,

$$avDO_2 \text{ (pulmonary bed)} = 12 \times 1.36\,(0.96 - 0.85) = 1.8$$

$$avDO_2 \text{ (systemic bed)} = 12 \times 1.36\,(0.96 - 0.61) = 5.7$$

Rearranging the formula for the respective vascular beds:

$$CO \text{ (systemic flow)} = \frac{VO_2}{avDO_2 \text{ (systemic bed)}}$$

$$CO \text{ (pulmonary flow)} = \frac{VO_2}{avDO_2 \text{ (pulmonary bed)}}$$

and therefore:

$$\frac{CO \text{ (systemic)}}{CO \text{ (pulmonary)}} = \frac{avDO_2 \text{ (pulmonary)}}{avDO_2 \text{ (systemic)}}$$

It can be seen that the ratio of systemic to pulmonary flow is equal to the ratio of the reciprocal arteriovenous oxygen differences. In this patient:

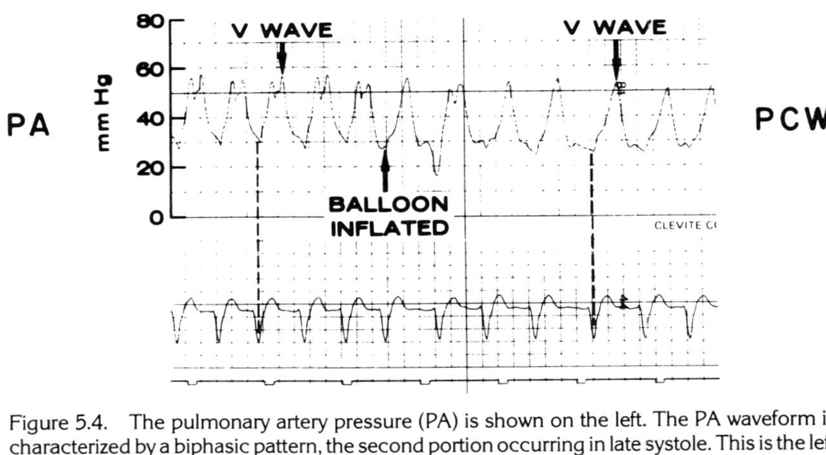

Figure 5.4. The pulmonary artery pressure (PA) is shown on the left. The PA waveform is characterized by a biphasic pattern, the second portion occurring in late systole. This is the left atrial V wave which is transmitted retrograde through the pulmonary veins and capillaries to the pulmonary artery. When the balloon is inflated, the pulmonary artery wedge pressure (PCW) is seen and reveals a giant V wave. Note that the V wave is further away from the QRS complex in the wedge position. When recorded from this position, the giant V wave is strongly suggestive of mitral regurgitation. If the giant V wave is not appreciated, the PCW waveform can be misinterpreted as a PA waveform. Under these circumstances, advancing the catheter further or leaving it in a distal position could lead to pulmonary artery rupture or pulmonary infarction. This same waveform observed from the right atrium would suggest tricuspid insufficiency. Reproduced from Forrester et al., 1976 (4) with permission.

$$\frac{\text{avDO}_2\ (\text{pulmonary})}{\text{avDO}_2\ (\text{systemic})} = \frac{1.8}{5.7} = \frac{\text{CO (systemic)}}{\text{CO (pulmonary)}}$$

pulmonary: systemic flow ratio is therefore 5.7:1.8, or about 3:1. With a pulmonary flow of 6 liters/min determined by the thermodilution method, systemic flow (cardiac output) in this patient was only 2 liters/min.

The patient was treated with dobutamine and nitroprusside, with reduction of shunting to 2:1 and elevation of systemic cardiac output to 4 liters/min. Cardiac catheterization demonstrated triple vessel coronary artery disease with total occlusion of the left anterior descending artery between the first and second septal perforating branches. A large portion of the anterior septal wall was dyskinetic, and global ejection fraction was 42%; both the septal defect and mitral regurgitation were confirmed angiographically. The patient underwent four-vessel coronary bypass, aneurysmectomy, patch repair of the ventricular septal defect (VSD) and replacement of the mitral valve with a porcine prosthesis. After 1 year of follow up, he remains a New York Heart Association (NYHA) Class II.

Discussion:

Cardiac rupture in the form of a ruptured portion of the papillary muscle or of the interventricular septum occurs in approximately 1% of patients with acute myocardial infarction. The usual clinical presentation includes auscultation of a new systolic murmur during the initial 2 weeks and a deteriorating hemodynamic status. The onset is often sudden, even cataclysmic, but may also occur over a matter of days. Although the location, quality, and radiation of the murmur often characterize the pathology, the auscultatory features may be ambiguous. Right heart catheterization establishes the diagnosis (12). The presence of "ventricularized" V waves in the wedge pressure almost invariably signals mitral regurgitation. Although mitral regurgitation is the most common cause of V waves, V waves are not extremely sensitive or specific for this diagnosis. In a recent study, 36% of patients with large V waves did not have significant mitral regurgitation and 32% of patients with severe regurgitation had only trivial V waves (13). Increased left atrial compliance may be associated with trivial V waves, despite severe mitral regurgitation, and patients with mitral obstruction, congestive heart failure, or ventricular septal defects may have large V waves in the absence of significant regurgitation (13). On the other hand, the presence of a step-up in oxygen saturation establishes the diagnosis of a ruptured interventricular septum and its absence effectively rules out this problem.

The present patient had evidence of a step-up in oxygen saturation and the diagnosis of an intracardiac shunt was made. The V waves were assumed to indicate that mitral regurgitation was also present. This was later confirmed angiographically. The V waves could have been secondary to the ventricular septal defect, but as noted above, mitral regurgitation is a more common cause for these findings.

PATIENT 4: VASODILATION/Charles L. Sprung

A 26-year-old man with a 10-year history of alcohol abuse was admitted for dyspnea. The patient was found to be in congestive heart failure and was treated with digoxin and furosemide. The patient improved symptomatically with this treatment. An echocardiogram revealed four-chamber enlargement, general hypokinesis, and an ejection fraction of 21%—findings consistent with a congestive cardiomyopathy. Several days later the patient developed severe respiratory distress. On physical examination the pulse was 120 beats/min, the blood pressure was 130/70 mm Hg, and the respiratory rate was 48 breaths/min. Jugular venous distension was present to the angle of the mandible at 45°. The lungs had bilateral rales up to the apices with dullness and decreased breath sounds at the bases. The PMI was at the 6th intercostal space at the anterior axillary line and a right ventricular heave was palpated. An S_3 and S_4 gallop were auscultated but a murmur was not heard. Abdominal exam revealed hepatosplenomegaly and diffuse voluntary guarding. Bilateral 3+ pedal edema was also noted. The electrocardiogram showed sinus tachycardia and nonspecific ST and T wave changes. The chest x-ray can be seen in Figure 5.5. The white blood count was 7,100/cu mm, the Hct was 34.2%, the BUN 46 mg/dl, and the creatinine 2.5 mg/dl. The arterial blood gas (FIO_2 - 0.35) was pH 7.34, pO_2 was 70 mm Hg, and pCO_2 was 21 mm Hg. Because of worsening pulmonary edema in the face of optimal digitalis therapy (digoxin level 1.9 mg/ml), pulmonary artery catheterization was performed for vasodilation. Initial hemodynamic data can be seen in Profile Chart 5.2, profile #1. Nitroprusside was begun and a repeat profile can be seen in Profile Chart 5.2, profile #2. Additional increases in nitroprusside, increased the cardiac output further as can be seen in profile #3.

Discussion

Chronic congestive heart failure secondary to ischemic or nonischemic heart disease has traditionally been treated with digitalis and diuretics. Unfortunately, many patients may have progressive left ventricular failure despite these medications. Further increases in digitalis and diuretics can cause toxicity and may be dangerous. Excessive diuretic therapy can decrease left ventricular filling pressures and decrease stroke volume. Over the last few years, vasodilator therapy has been used for the treatment of refractory heart failure. The long-term results of vasodilator therapy are still unknown. Despite the apparent clinical and hemodynamic improvements, the effect of this treatment on morbidity and mortality has not been established.

Patients with cardiac failure may have symptoms of backward failure and congestion (dyspnea, orthopnea, etc.), forward failure and hypoperfusion (weakness, fatigue, etc.), or both. An increase in systemic vascular resistance typically occurs in left ventricular failure. This may be secondary to an increased sympathetic nervous system activity to maintain flow and/or increased secretion of renin and salt and water retention. Vasodilators can decrease arterial impedance and/or increase venous capacitance. An increase in the compliance of the large arteries or a decrease in the arteriolar resistance will decrease arterial impedance and systemic vascular resis-

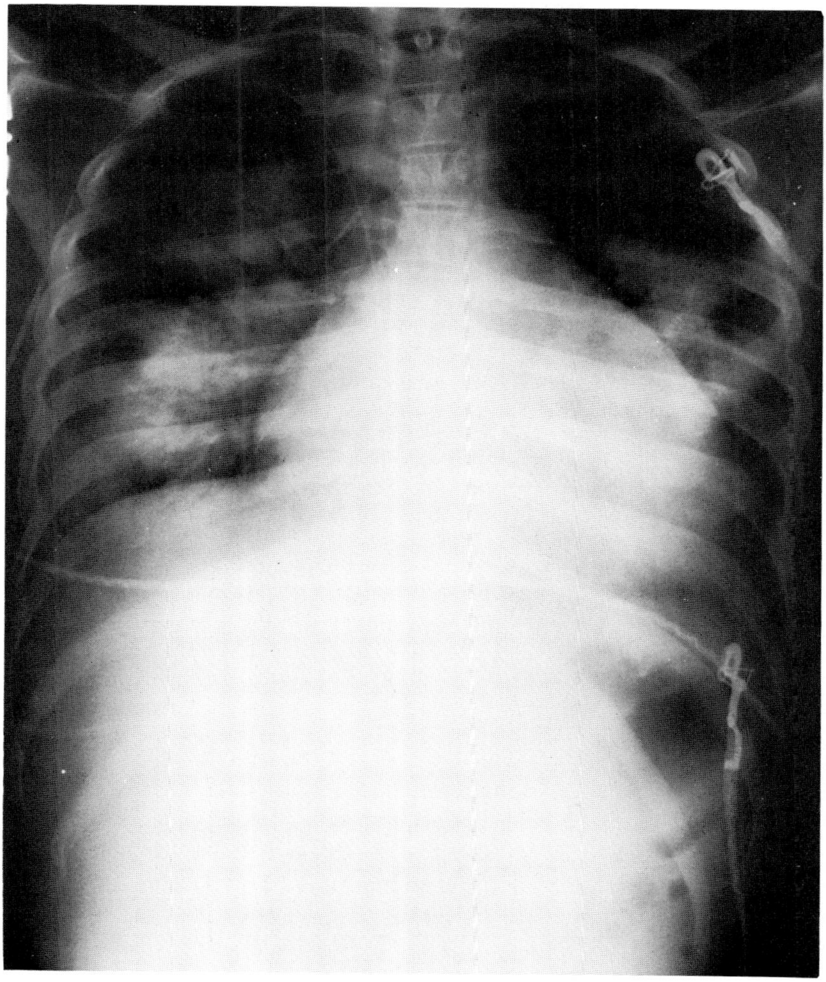

Figure 5.5. A chest roentgenogram demonstrating cardiomegaly and severe pulmonary edema.

tance. As vascular resistance is decreased by vasodilators, systemic arterial pressure decreases unless there is a corresponding increase in cardiac output (BP = SVR × CO). In the normal heart, a reduction in outflow resistance is not accompanied by an increase in stroke volume, and blood pressure may fall with vasodilation. The decrease in systemic pressure may be minimized, however, by the reflex tachycardia which usually increases cardiac output. On the other hand, patients with myocardial dysfunction increase their stroke volume in response to a decrease in outflow resistance. This increase in cardiac output compensates for the decrease in systemic vascular resistance and blood pressure is affected minimally (Figure 5.6) (14).

Profile Chart 5.2. Cardiopulmonary profile of patient undergoing vasodilation

Enter: Date/time:	# 1	# 2	# 3
Cardiac output (CO)	3.16	4.0	5.25
Systolic blood pressure (SBP)	138	135	130
Diastolic blood pressure (DBP)	85	80	67
Mean arterial pressure (MAP)	103	98	88
Heart rate (HR)	112	115	112
Mean pulmonary artery pressure (MPAP)	35	32	25
Pulmonary artery wedge pressure (PWP)	25	20	14
Central venous pressure (CVP)	18	17	12
Body surface area (BSA)	1.7	1.7	1.7
Data:			
Stroke volume (SV)	28.2	34.8	46.9
Cardiac index (CI)	1.9	2.4	3.1
Stroke index (SI)	16.6	20.5	27.6
Right ventricular stroke work (RVSW)	4	4	5
RVSW/CVP ratio	0.22	0.24	0.42
Left ventricular stroke work (LVSW)	18	22	47
LVSW/PWP ratio	0.72	1.1	3.4
Systemic vascular resistance (SVR)	2149	1617	1157
Pulmonary vascular resistance (PVR)	253	240	167
Enter:			
Hemoglobin (Hgb)	11.0	11.0	11.0
FIO_2	0.35	0.35	0.35
$PaCO_2$	21	31	30
PaO_2	70	60	74
SaO_2	0.92	0.90	0.95
PvO_2	21	25	33
SvO_2	0.29	0.42	0.61
Data:			
Capillary O_2 content (CcO_2)	15.7	15.6	15.6
Mixed venous O_2 content (CvO_2)	4.4	6.4	9.2
Arterial O_2 content (CaO_2)	14.0	13.7	14.4
Arteriovenous O_2 content difference ($avDO_2$)	9.6	7.3	5.2
O_2 delivery	442	548	756
O_2 consumption (VO_2)	303	292	273
O_2 utilization ratio	0.69	0.53	0.36
Intrapulmonary shunt (Qs/Qt)	0.15	0.21	0.19
PaO_2/FIO_2	200	171	211
Vasopressors or vasodilators (μ/k/m)	—	Nipride 0.5	Nipride 1.5

Venodilation causes a redistribution of the central intravascular blood volume to the periphery. This decreases pulmonary artery wedge pressure and relieves the symptoms of congestion. In a normal heart with a steep Starling curve, a precipitous decrease in PWP decreases stroke volume. The patient with myocardial dysfunction, in contrast, operates on a flat Starling curve and a decrease in PWP might not affect stroke volume appreciably (Figure 5.7). Therefore, vasodilation, which may be deleterious in a patient with a normal heart because of a decreased stroke volume with arterial dilation and a possible further decreased stroke volume with venodilation, may be extremely beneficial to the patient with myocardial dysfunction. The patient with left ventricular failure will increase stroke volume in response to arterial vasodilation and will usually not decrease stroke volume with venodilation. In addition, tachycardia does not occur to the same extent in these patients as it does in patients without heart disease.

The majority of patients in the United States are probably placed on vasodilator therapy without the aid of hemodynamic monitoring. It is certainly advisable, however, to use hemodynamic monitoring to vasodilate patients with low blood pressure or patients whose cardiac indices are dependent on a certain left ventricular filling pressure. In addition, hemodynamic monitoring enables the physician to titrate the vasodilator for a maximum hemodynamic response which might not be possible by clinical means. After pulmonary artery and systemic arterial catheterization, an intravenous vasodilator with rapid onset and short duration is begun. These vasodilators include nitroprusside, phentolamine, trimethaphan, and nitroglycerin. Sodium nitroprusside dilates vessels in both the arterial and venous circuits. Doses range from 15 to 400 μg/minute. Side effects include hypotension from overdosage (uncommon and readily reversible by discontinuing the nitroprusside infusion) and thiocyanate toxicity after prolonged administration. Phentolamine is an alpha-adrenergic receptor antagonist and primarily affects the arterial vasculature. Doses range from 0.2 to 2.0 mg/minute. Nitroprusside is more commonly used because of the greater incidence of tachycardia with phentolamine and the added expense of phentolamine. Trimethaphan is a ganglionic blocking agent which predominantly effects the venous capacitance vessels as opposed to the arterial vessels. Because of severe orthostatic hypotension and tachyphylaxis, which develops quickly, trimethaphan has not been widely used. Nitroglycerin predominantly affects the venous system, as compared to the arterial system. Nitroglycerin may also have additional antianginal effects in patients with ischemic heart disease.

Most patients with severe pump failure unresponsive to digitalis and diuretics require a decrease in the elevated PWP and an increase in the reduced cardiac output. Therefore, nitroprusside which can accomplish both of these goals is typically used. As nitroprusside is slowly titrated up-

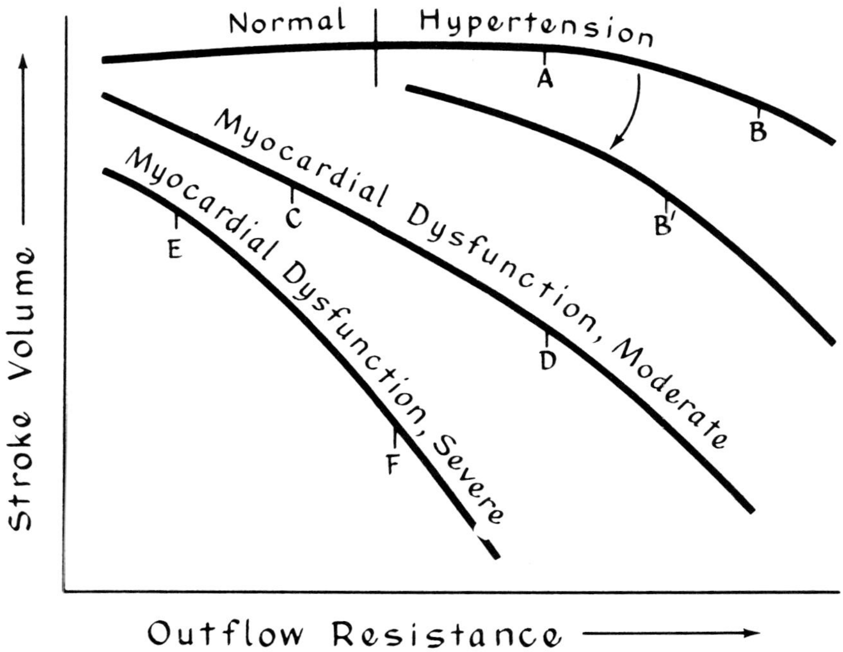

Figure 5.6. The relationship of left ventricular stroke volume to systemic outflow resistance in normal and diseased hearts. Different curves represent the severity of myocardial disease. In the normal heart, a rise in resistance results in hypertension since cardiac output remains relatively constant. Heart failure in a hypertensive patient could result from high resistance and normal function *(B)* or high resistance and depressed ventricular function *(B')*. With severe myocardial dysfunction (lower two curves), blood pressure is no longer directly determined by resistance because stroke volume and resistance are inversely related. Therefore, arterial pressure may be similar at points E and F despite large differences in cardiac output and resistance. Reproduced from Cohn and Franciosa, 1977 (14) with permission.

ward, the PWP and SVR decrease. Blood pressure remains unchanged secondary to an increase in cardiac output. As vasodilation progresses, the PWP and SVR fall further. Cardiac output continues to increase but will eventually level off and remain the same despite additional vasodilation. If the PWP falls too low, cardiac output will decrease. This can be avoided by closely watching the PWP (or the pulmonary artery diastolic pressure if it correlates with the PWP) together with cardiac output measurements. If the PWP falls to a low level (typically 10-15 mm Hg or less), volume infusions can increase the PWP and enable continued vasodilation; this is especially helpful in patients with severe prerenal azotemia. After SVR and PWP decrease and cardiac output no longer increases, the blood pressure may begin to fall. It is at this point that vasodilation should be discontinued. Further vasodilation may lead to a further decrease in PWP, SVR, and car-

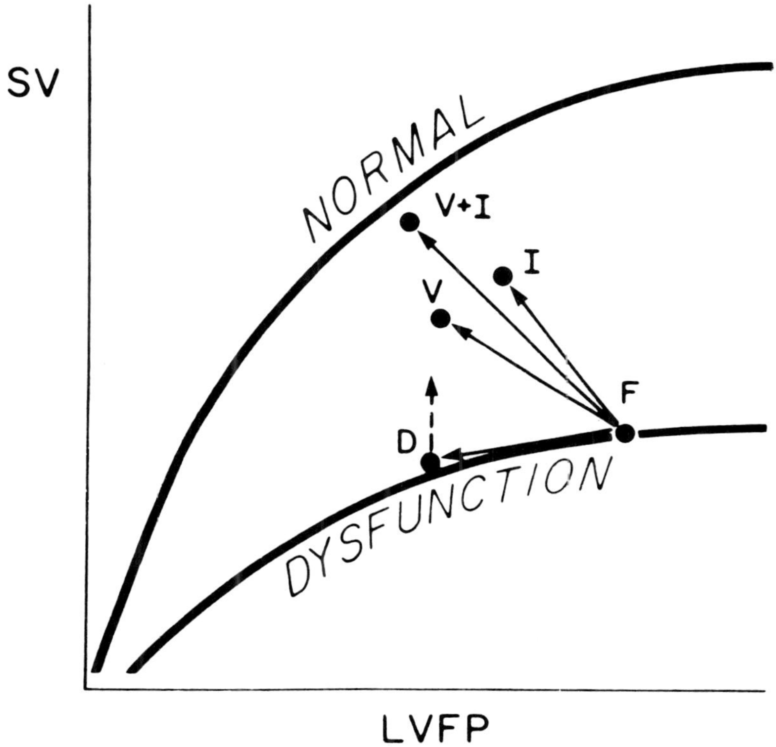

Figure 5.7. A Frank-Starling left ventricular function curve relating left ventricular filling pressure (LVFP) to stroke volume (SV). The depressed curve found in patients with myocardial dysfunction can be shifted toward normal by inotropic (I) or vasodilator (V) drugs. The effects of these drugs are complementary when used together (V + I). Note that diuretics (D) usually decrease filling pressure (F) without increasing cardiac output. If LVFP falls too low cardiac output may actually decrease. Reproduced from Cohn and Franciosa, 1977 (14) with permission.

diac output and cause a precipitous drop in blood pressure. Vasodilation should, therefore, only be attempted in patients with adequate left ventricular filling pressures.

As noted in Figure 5.6, the greatest response to vasodilation can be expected in patients with the highest vascular resistance. Once invasive hemodynamic monitoring has been performed, cardiac function should be maximized by vasodilation. This is preferable to decreasing PWP and increasing cardiac output minimally to merely improve symptomatology. After a maximal cardiac output has been determined, oral vasodilators can be added as the intravenous vasodilator is weaned off. The oral agents include the nitrates, hydralazine, prazosin, and minoxidil. Nitrates predominately affect the venous bed, whereas hydralazine and minoxidil affect the arterial bed. Prazosin affects the arterial and venous circuit. Therefore, the oral equivalent of nitroprusside is prazosin or a combination of nitrates and hydralazine. In the future, angiotension-converting enzyme inhibitors and calcium channel blockers may also be used more commonly for vasodilation.

The present patient had a decreased cardiac index, stroke volume index (SVI), LVSW, and an increased PWP and SVR. The SVR was elevated and the decreased myocardial parameters were especially impressive for a 26-year-old man. Because of these contractility difficulties, the patient had a low pvO_2 and oxygen transport, and a markedly increased $avDO_2$, O_2 utilization ratio, and oxygen consumption. The below-normal hemoglobin and arterial oxygen tensions compounded the problems. With initial vasodilation with nitroprusside (Profile Chart 5.2, profile #2), the cardiac index (CI), SVI, and LVSW increased and the PWP and SVR decreased. With these changes, the pvO_2 and O_2 transport began to increase and the $avDO_2$, O_2 utilization ratio, and O_2 consumption decreased. With further nitroprusside therapy (profile #3), a further improvement in cardiac function and oxygen supply occurred. Note that the PWP decreased to 14 mm Hg and the SVR decreased to 1,158 dyne·sec·cm^{-5}. Further vasodilation without adequate filling pressures might be dangerous. Further vasodilation after increasing the PWP did not provide a further improvement in myocardial function. Thereafter, the patient received prazosin (while the nitroprusside was slowly decreased) until similar hemodynamic results as found in profile #3 were obtained with oral therapy.

PATIENT 5: SEPTIC SHOCK/Charles L. Sprung

A 42-year-old man presented with a 1-day history of fever (temperature of 104° F), chills, nausea, vomiting, diarrhea, and midepigastric pain. The patient had polycythemia vera for 9 years treated with ^{32}P and leukeran.

Vital signs revealed a blood pressure of 70 systolic; pulse, 120 beats/min; temperature, 101° F; and respiratory rate, 30 breaths/min. The rest of the physical exam was positive for dry mucous membranes, a grade II/VI systolic ejection murmur at the left sternal border, mild epigastric tenderness, a liver palpable 3 cm below the right costal margin, and a spleen 8 cm below the left costal margin. The patient was alert and oriented to time, place, and person.

Laboratory data included a white blood cell count of 37,600/cu mm with 85% blasts; Hct, 29.1%; platelets, 80,000/cu mm; sodium, 132 mEq/liter; potassium, 3.1 mEq/liter; chloride, 104mEq/liter; carbon dioxide, 16 mEq/liter; BUN, 42 mg/dl; creatinine, 3.4 mg/dl; and colloid osmotic pressure, 15.9 mm Hg. The arterial blood gas on room air was pH 7.38; pO_2, 52 mm Hg; and $p\,CO_2$, 20 mm Hg. Chest roentgenogram revealed a normal sized heart and no infiltrates. The urinalysis and spinal fluid examinations were negative.

Hospital Course

The patient was presumed to have sepsis and started on ticarcillin, cephalothin, and tobramycin. Volume resuscitation with several liters of normal saline increased the blood pressure to 110/60 mm Hg and the CVP from 8 to 14 cm H_2O. The patient did well for approximately 12 hours. On morning rounds the patient was noted to be lethargic and tachypneic. His BP was 65/40 mm Hg; pulse, 110 beats/min; respiratory rate, 40 breaths/min; and CVP, 19 cm H_2O. The patient now had jugular venous distension, bilateral rales on chest examination, and an S_3 gallop. The patient was immediately begun on dopamine 5 μg/kg/min which increased the BP to 90/50 mm Hg.

Pulmonary artery catheterization was performed and the initial hemodynamic profile can be seen in Profile Chart 5.3. At this time, the patient was on 10 μg/kg min of dopamine to maintain an acceptable BP with signs of adequate perfusion. *Staphylococcus aureus* was cultured from the patient's blood. Despite antibiotics, the patient developed disseminated intravascular coagulation, worsening shock requiring higher doses of dopamine (27 μg/kg/min), and renal failure. A subsequent hemodynamic profile is shown in Profile Chart 5.3, profile #2.

Discussion

Septic shock is characterized by inadequate tissue perfusion. It usually is secondary to gram-negative bacillary infection but may follow gram-positive infections, also. Endotoxin induces a sympathetic (alpha-adrenergic) effect on small blood vessels which causes intense arteriolar and venous constriction. Tissue anoxia and subsequent acidosis lead to relaxation of arteriolar sphincters, despite continued venous constriction. This leads to pooling of blood in the capillary bed. Increased hydrostatic pressure pushes fluid from the intravascular space into the interstitial space. In addition, bradykinin, a potent vasodilator, is activated and increases capillary permeability which causes a leakage of plasma proteins into the interstitium. These factors cause a dramatic decrease in circulating blood volume. If inadequate perfusion of the vital organs persists, metabolic (lactic) acidosis, severe organ damage, and finally irreversible shock occur. Because there is no clinical marker to determine when irreversible shock occurs, all patients with shock must be treated aggressively so that the shock state can be reversed quickly before irreversible shock ensues.

With an understanding of the above pathophysiologic mechanisms, it is not surprising that the initial therapy of septic shock is volume resuscitation. Fluid boluses are given over 10–15 minute intervals. If several of these infusions are inadequate to reverse the shock state, CVP or pulmonary artery catheterization is performed and the boluses are continued under close pressure monitoring. As left ventricular filling pressure is increased, the cardiac output increases. Because blood pressure is the product of cardiac output and systemic vascular resistance, an increase in cardiac output is often followed by an increase in blood pressure and reversal of shock. Volume is infused to increase the pulmonary artery wedge pressure and cardiac output while the PWP is closely observed so that pulmonary edema does not occur. As the PWP increases with fluid therapy, one can serially measure cardiac output and construct a Starling curve for each individual

Profile Chart 5.3. Cardiopulmonary profile of patient with septic shock

Enter: **Date/time:**	# 1	# 2	# 3
Cardiac output (CO)	11.7	6.7	6.7
Systolic blood pressure (SBP)	81	99	99
Diastolic blood pressure (DBP)	34	40	40
Mean arterial pressure (MAP)	49	59	59
Heart rate (HR)	148	134	134
Mean pulmonary artery pressure (MPAP)	25	26	26
Pulmonary artery wedge pressure (PWP)	12	19	19
Central venous pressure (CVP)	8	15	15
Body surface area (BSA)	2.02	2.02	2.02
Data:			
Stroke volume (SV)	79.1	50.0	50.0
Cardiac index (CI)	5.8	3.3	3.3
Stroke index (SI)	39.1	24.8	24.8
Right ventricular stroke work (RVSW)	9	4	4
RVSW/CVP ratio	1.13	0.27	0.27
Left ventricular stroke work (LVSW)	20	13	13
LVSW/PWP ratio	1.67	0.68	0.68
Systemic vascular resistance (SVR)	280	525	525
Pulmonary vascular resistance (PVR)	89	83	83
Enter:			
Hemoglobin (Hgb)	9.3	9.8	9.8
FIO_2	0.5	0.4	0.4
$PaCO_2$	37	26	26
PaO_2	80	82	82
SaO_2	0.92	0.93	0.94
PvO_2	43	31	31
SvO_2	0.71	0.46	0.50
DATA:			
Capillary O_2 content (CcO_2)	13.5	14.1	14.1
Mixed venous O_2 content (CvO_2)	9.1	6.2	6.8
Arterial O_2 content (CaO_2)	11.8	12.6	12.7
Arteriovenous O_2 content difference ($avDO_2$)	2.7	6.4	5.9
O_2 delivery	1381	844	851
O_2 consumption (VO_2)	316	429	395
O_2 utilization ratio	0.23	0.51	0.46
Intrapulmonary shunt (Qs/Qt)	0.39	0.19	0.19
PaO_2/FIO_2	160	205	205
Vasopressors or vasodilators (μ/k/m)	Dopa 10	Dopa 27	Dopa 27

patient. If maximum cardiac function (cardiac output, stroke index, and stroke work) occurs at normal filling pressures, there is no need to increase PWP further and increase the risk of pulmonary edema. In fact, there are preliminary data to suggest that patients with septic shock have optimal cardiac function at normal (12 mm Hg) rather than high (16 mm Hg) PWP (15). If an optimal PWP is obtained and the patient remains in shock, a vasopressor (usually dopamine) is started. Dopamine is titrated to a dose which will increase blood pressure and improve perfusion. In most patients this constitutes a systolic blood pressure of 90-100 mm Hg or a mean blood pressure of 60 mm Hg. The ideal blood pressure, however, is that pressure which improves and maintains adequate perfusion—urine output, mental status, and so on.

The appropriate fluid to use in patients with shock has been hotly and vociferously debated (16-21). This has become known as the colloid-crystalloid controversy. Both sides of the issue agree that the objective of treatment is to rapidly achieve hemodynamic stability and tissue perfusion by increasing blood volume, blood flow, and oxygen delivery. There are advantages and disadvantages to each of the available solutions. Colloids (albumin, dextrans, hydroxyethyl starch, and blood) are expensive, are more effective in restoring blood volume, blood pressure, cardiac output, and oxygen transport, and do not produce overexpansion of interstitial water content. Crystalloids (Ringer's Lactate, saline, and glucose solutions) are cheap, can restore blood volume, blood pressure, cardiac output, and oxygen transport when given in sufficient quantities, and expand interstitial volume more than they increase plasma volume. Both sides have claimed a lesser incidence of pulmonary complications using their preferred solutions.

We have been involved in the study of colloid osmotic pressure and its importance in the development of pulmonary edema. Movement of fluid into the pulmonary interstitium and alveoli is a function not only of the intravascular hydrostatic pressure pushing fluid from the intravascular space into the interstitium but also of plasma colloid osmotic pressure which draws fluid from the interstitium into the vascular space. Patients may, therefore, be in pulmonary edema with a normal or "high normal" PWP if the colloid osmotic pressure (COP) is decreased. Rackow et al. (22) have shown that patients with decreased COP-PWP gradients (less than 4 mm Hg) have clinical evidence of pulmonary edema whereas those patients with normal gradients do not (Figure 5.8). We have preferred to use colloid rather than crystalloid solutions for shock because the COP can be maintained or increased as the PWP is increased. If crystalloid solutions are used, the COP will decrease significantly (because of the dilution of plasma proteins) at the same time the PWP is increasing. Colloids are especially useful in patients with severe shock who require large and rapid increases in blood pressure.

The hemodynamic responses in patients with bacterial shock have varied (23). Shock is usually accompanied by a profound decrease in blood pressure but the cardiac output may be increased, normal, or decreased. The early stage of septic shock is characteristically hyperdynamic with an increase in cardiac output and a decrease in systemic vascular resistance. Significant arteriovenous shunting occurs around capillary beds. In addition, cells may be unable to utilize available oxygen. The net result is tissue anoxia and lactic acidosis, despite a decreased arteriovenous oxygen difference. Progression of the shock state leads to a hypodynamic response—a decreased cardiac output and increased systemic vascular resistance. Several studies have reported different hemodynamic findings. These differences are most likely related to concomitant hypovolemia, underlying heart disease or liver cirrhosis, the causative organism, and the duration of shock. The mortality of patients in septic shock is inversely proportional to the cardiac output. The likelihood of survival is much greater when the car-

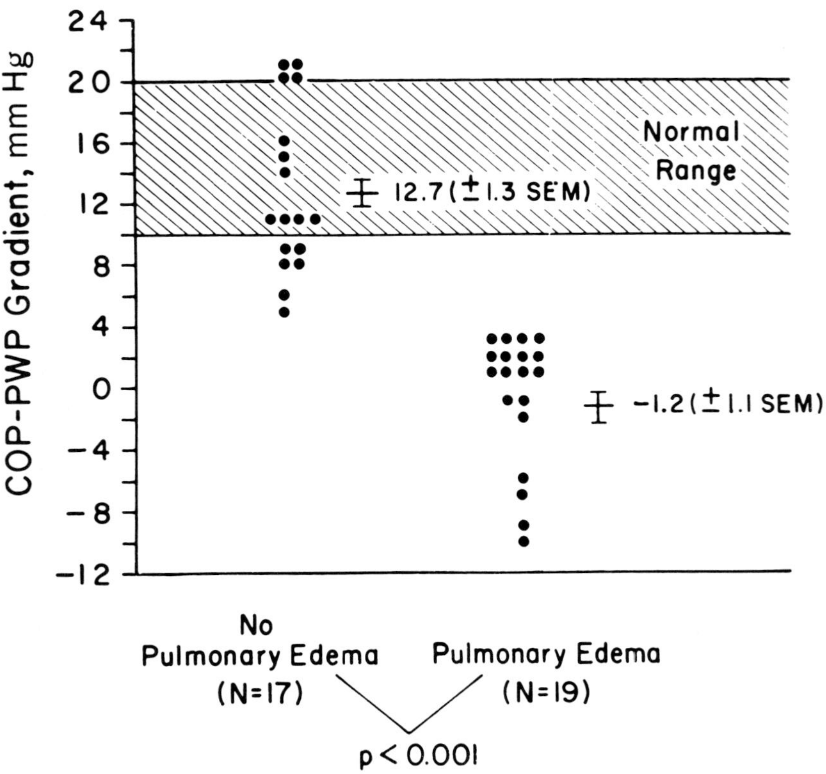

Figure 5.8. Colloid osmotic pressure (COP)—pulmonary artery wedge pressure (PWP) gradients and the presence or absence of pulmonary edema. A COP-PWP gradient of 4 mm Hg separated those patients with pulmonary edema from those without pulmonary edema very well. Reproduced from Rackow et al., 1977 (22) with permission.

diac output is normal or increased (23). Other prognostic indicators of the severity of shock and mortality include lactate levels and pulmonary hypertension (manifested by a pulmonary artery diastolic pressure-pulmonary artery wedge pressure gradient $>$ 5 mm Hg) (23, 24).

The present patient developed acute myelogenous leukemia (AML) after treatment for his polycythemia vera. Other known predisposing factors for the development of septic shock include: diabetes mellitus, cirrhosis, lymphoma, disseminated carcinoma, childbirth, surgical procedures, previous infections of the urinary, biliary, or gastrointestinal tract, and disorders requiring immunosuppressive therapy. Shock occurs in approximately 40% of patients with gram-negative bacteremia and early appropriate antibiotic therapy can reduce the frequency of shock by one half (25).

The present patient responded well to fluid therapy for his initial hypotensive episode which was most likely secondary to hypovolemia. This was accomplished quickly and the patient did not require pulmonary artery catheterization. Several hours later the patient again developed hypotension; this episode was accompanied by signs of congestive heart failure and the patient therefore underwent pulmonary artery catheterization.

The initial hemodynamic profile (see Profile Chart 5.3, profile #1) demonstrated a hyperdynamic response with a markedly elevated cardiac output and a decreased systemic vascular resistance. These alterations were accompanied by an elevated mixed venous oxygen tension and decreased $avDO_2$ which is typical of the shunting found in septic shock. Despite this hyperdynamic activity, most patients with bacteremic shock have a markedly increased heart rate, and therefore, have a decreased stroke volume index and stroke work. The patient also had evidence of arterial hypoxemia and an increased pulmonary shunt (Qs/Qt). These latter abnormalities have been demonstrated in septic shock and are thought to result from an abnormal pattern of gas distribution with closure of alveoli and/or airways, an abnormal pattern of blood flow distribution in the lung with closure of capillaries, or an increase in pulmonary extravascular water with interstitial or alveolar edema (26). The present patient's hypoxemia, however, was worse than is usually found in septic shock.

The patient underwent continued volume resuscitation to increase cardiac output and decrease the amount of dopamine he was receiving, but as the PWP increased, cardiac output and other cardiac indices did not change. Thereafter, the PWP was maintained at approximately 12 mm Hg. This was the PWP with the maximum cardiac output and stroke work and approximately 4 mm Hg less than the COP. Despite appropriate antibiotic and other treatment modalities, the patient's shock was not reversed and continued to worsen. A repeat hemodynamic profile (see Profile Chart 5.3., profile #2) a day later revealed that the cardiac output, stroke index, and stroke work decreased despite an increased PWP and a higher concentration of dopamine. The systemic vascular resistance was higher than the previous value but remained low—most likely due to arteriovenous shunting as evidenced by the widened pulse pressure. This indicated more of a hypodynamic response possibly secondary to decreased myocardial contractility. The oxygen delivery was decreased and was no longer adequate to support the increased metabolic and circulatory demands of the body. Because of this, the mixed venous oxygen tension decreased and the $avDO_2$, the lactate concentration, and the oxygen utilization ratio were extremely elevated. The oxygen consumption remained excessively elevated evidenced by the marked increase in $avDO_2$. These hemodynamic findings are typically noted in the preterminal period of patients with septic shock.

Profile #3 contains the same data as profile #2, except that the calculated venous oxygen saturation (0.50) is substituted for the actual measured saturation (0.46) of profile #2. By comparing the measured and calculated saturations, one can get an idea of any shift in the oxygen dissociation curve. In this case, the patient had a lactic acidosis and the lower measured saturation signified a shift of the curve to the right. Therefore, more oxygen is available to the tissues and the $avDO_2$ is higher.

The patient's shock progressed further such that his blood pressure could not be maintained with dopamine or norepinephrine. He died soon thereafter, and on postmortem examination, was found to have acute myelogenous leukemia and endocarditis of the tricuspid and aortic valves.

PATIENT 6: ADULT RESPIRATORY DISTRESS SYNDROME/ Charles L. Sprung

A 50-year-old man with previous alcoholic liver disease was admitted for upper gastrointestinal bleeding. The patient complained of sharp mid-epigastric pain for 3 days and vomiting bright red blood for 2 days. The patient took aspirin and Alka Seltzer twice daily for the pain. In addition, the patient noticed an increasing abdominal girth over the past 3 weeks.

Physical examination revealed blood pressure, 100/70 mm Hg and pulse, 100 beats/min, which changed to 85/70 mm Hg and 120 beats/min, respectively, upon sitting; respirations, 18 breaths/min; and temperature, 99.6° F. Pulmonary and heart examination were normal. The abdominal exam revealed slight tenderness in the midepigastrium and tense ascites. The liver and spleen could not be palpated. Extremities were positive for 4+ pedal edema and palmar erythema.

Laboratory data included a white blood cell count of 6600/cu mm; Hct, 35.4% which decreased to 26.2% after 1½ liters of normal saline; platelets, 102,000/cu mm; prothrombin time, 16.9/12.9 seconds; partial thromboplastin time, 40 seconds; bilirubin, 1.5 mg/dl; serum glutamic oxalacetic transaminase (SGOT), 91 mU/ml; alkaline phosphatase, 157 mU/ml; lactic dehydrogenase (LDH) 247 mU/ml; BUN, 17 mg/dl; creatinine, 0.9 mg/dl; amylase, 95 units/dl; total protein, 6.1 grams/dl; and albumin, 1.6 grams/dl.

A nasogastric tube was placed and bright red blood with clots were aspirated. After continuous ice saline lavage, the bleeding stopped. The patient received 2 units of packed red blood cells and 3 units of fresh frozen plasma. The patient remained stable through the night with a Hct of 30%. Endoscopy in the morning revealed an esophageal ulcer and no varices. One hour later the patient vomited 3 liters of blood. Blood pressure was 60 mm Hg systolic which increased to 100/60 mm Hg after two units of whole blood and saline. Nasogastric lavage was started again. Celiac and selective left gastric angiography did not reveal a bleeding site or varices, but embolization of the left gastric artery was performed. Bleeding stopped after the procedure.

After 24 hours the patient complained of dyspnea. Physical exam demonstrated bilateral rales and wheezing. An arterial blood gas (5 liter nasal cannula) revealed: pH, 7.35; pO_2, 42 mm Hg; and pCO_2, 43 mm Hg. The patient was intubated shortly thereafter for severe hypoxia despite increasing inspired concentrations of oxygen and because of CO_2 retention. Immediately after intubation, red frothy edema fluid poured out of the endotracheal tube. The serum colloid osmotic pressure was 14.4 mm Hg, whereas the colloid osmotic pressure of the pulmonary edema fluid was 10.8 mm Hg. The edema fluid to serum colloid osmotic pressure ratio was therefore 75%. Pulmonary artery catheterization was performed to evaluate the possibility of volume overload and to help manage the required high levels of positive end-expiratory pressure. The cardiopulmonary changes which occurred with increasing levels of PEEP can be seen in Profile Chart 5.4.

Profile Chart 5.4. Cardiopulmonary profile of a patient with ARDS

Enter:	**Date/time:**	# 1	# 2	# 3	# 4
Cardiac output (CO)		6.8	6.4	5.5	6.7
Systolic blood pressure (SBP)		100	102	90	102
Diastolic blood pressure (DBP)		55	48	40	52
Mean arterial pressure (MAP)		70	66	57	71
Heart rate (HR)		132	128	140	132
Mean pulmonary artery pressure (MPAP)		27	30	26	26
Pulmonary artery wedge pressure (PWP)		6	12	16	13
Central venous pressure (CVP)		12	13	18	15
Body surface area (BSA)		1.7	1.7	1.7	1.7
Data:					
Stroke volume (SV)		51.5	50.0	39.3	50.8
Cardiac index (CI)		4.0	3.8	3.2	3.9
Stroke index (SI)		30.3	29.4	23.1	29.9
Right ventricular stroke work (RVSW)		6	7	3	4
RVSW/CVP ratio		0.50	0.54	0.17	0.27
Left ventricular stroke work (LVSW)		26	22	13	24
LVSW/PWP ratio		4.33	1.83	0.81	1.85
Systemic vascular resistance (SVR)		682	662	567	668
Pulmonary vascular resistance (PVR)		247	225	145	155

Profile Chart 5.4. (Continued)

Enter: Date/time:	# 1	# 2	# 3	# 4
Hemoglobin (Hgb)	13.0	13.0	11.0	10.5
FIO_2	0.8	0.7	0.7	0.7
$PaCO_2$	29	32	31	31
PaO_2	72	64	62	102
SaO_2	0.93	0.92	0.90	0.95
$P\bar{v}O_2$	32	34	32	37
$S\bar{v}O_2$	0.59	0.65	0.60	0.71
Data:				
Capillary O_2 content (CcO_2)	19.3	19.1	16.4	15.7
Mixed venous O_2 content ($C\bar{v}O_2$)	10.5	11.6	9.1	10.2
Arterial O_2 content (CaO_2)	16.7	16.5	13.7	13.9
Arteriovenous O_2 content difference ($avDO_2$)	6.2	4.9	4.6	3.7
O_2 delivery	1136	1056	754	931
O_2 consumption (VO_2)	422	314	253	248
O_2 utilization ratio	0.37	0.30	0.34	0.27
Intrapulmonary shunt (Qs/Qt)	0.30	0.35	0.37	0.33
PaO_2/FIO_2	90	91	89	146
Vasopressors or vasodilators (μ/k/m)	—	—	—	Dopa 5
PEEP	5	10	15	20
Respirator rate	2	2	2	2
Tidal volume	900	900	900	900
PIP	70	65	64	60

Discussion

Over the last 20 years, improvements in medical and surgical care have allowed patients with trauma or life threatening diseases to survive long enough to develop the nonspecific response of the lung to injury, noncardiogenic pulmonary edema. The adult respiratory distress syndrome (ARDS) is an extreme form of noncardiogenic pulmonary edema. The clinical features include acute respiratory distress, marked dyspnea and tachypnea, cyanosis, severe hypoxemia refractory to oxygen therapy, and diffuse bilateral pulmonary infiltrates. Pulmonary capillary hydrostatic pressures are usually normal. Alveolar filling or closure leads to a reduced functional residual capacity, decreased pulmonary compliance, intrapulmonary right-to-left shunting, and an increased alveolar to arterial oxygen tension gradient. A high index of suspicion must be present when caring for patients with any one of the many clinical conditions associated with the development of ARDS (Table 5.2).

An understanding of ARDS can be appreciated by a knowledge of the pathophysiology of edema formation. The Starling equation is often used to explain these concepts:

$$Q = K_f [(P_c - P_{is}) - \sigma_f (\pi_c - \pi_{is})]$$

where Q is the net transvascular flow of fluid, K_f is the filtration coefficient, P is the hydrostatic pressure in the capillary (P_c) and in the interstitial space (P_{is}), σ_f is the reflection coefficient which is a measure of the tendency of a membrane to restrict molecules, and π is the colloid osmotic pressure in the capillary (π_c) and in the interstitial space (π_{is}). Thus, there are four pressures, a hydrostatic pair and an osmotic pair. The principal force is the capillary hydrostatic pressure (P_c), which tends to increase filtration of fluid from the capillary into the interstitial space. Clinically, the pulmonary artery wedge pressure is used to evaluate hydrostatic pressures. Normal pressures are 5 to 15 mm Hg. The capillary colloid osmotic pressure (π_c) tends to draw fluid from the interstitial space into the intravascular space. The normal serum colloid osmotic pressure in ambulatory patients is approximately 25 mm Hg. Interstitial colloid osmotic pressure (π_{is}) is approximately two-thirds of the plasma value and tends to cause fluid movement from the intravascular to the interstitial space. Interstitial hydrostatic pressure (P_{is}) values are controversial but many investigators consider them to be negative. The filtration of fluid depends on the sum of these opposing pressures and the filtration and reflection coefficients. Normally, there is a small net outward filtration of fluid from the pulmonary capillaries which is returned to the vasculature by the lymphatics. When the filtration coefficient is increased, as occurs with increased capillary permeability, filtration may increase despite normal capillary hydrostatic pressure. Under these circumstances, the osmotic pressure differences become less significant.

The major causes of pulmonary edema are increased pulmonary capillary pressure, decreased colloid osmotic pressure, altered permeability, and lymphatic insufficiency. Increased hydrostatic pressure secondary to cardiac failure is the most common cause of pulmonary edema. Decreased colloid osmotic pressure (π_c) may be secondary to the hypoproteinemia of malabsorption, malnutrition, renal or hepatic disease, infusion of large volumes of crystalloid solutions, and severe bleeding. Patients with reduced plasma colloid osmotic pressure may develop pulmonary edema at normal hydrostatic pressure (1, 22). Altered permeability occurs because of damage to alveolar epithelial or pulmonary capillary endothelial cells. Lymphatic insufficiency may also be a cause of pulmonary edema because the lymphatics represent a valuable safety mechanism for the prevention of edema

Table 5.2. Conditions associated with the adult respiratory distress syndrome

I. Shock (Shock Lung)
   A. Hypovolemic
   B. Endotoxic

II. Central nervous system insults (neurogenic pulmonary edema)
   A. Head trauma
   B. Convulsions
   C. Cerebrovascular accidents
   D. Neoplasms
   E. Increased cerebrospinal fluid pressure
   F. Hanging

III. Direct pulmonary insults
   A. Chest trauma
   B. Viral or bacterial pneumonia
   C. Fat embolism
   D. Aspiration pneumonia
   E. Near drowning
   F. Radiation pneumonia
   G. Pulmonary burn or smoke inhalation
   H. Chemical lung burn (NO_2, CL_2, NH_3, phosgene, cadmium)
   I. Oxygen toxicity
   J. Diffuse infiltrative disease: tuberculous pneumonitis, lymphagitic spread of cancer to lung

IV. Miscellaneous
   A. Drugs: Heroin, methadone, propoxyphene, barbiturates, colchicine, acetylsalicylic acid, ethchlorvynol, busulfan, bleomycin, cyclophosphamide, paraquat
   B. Cardiopulmonary bypass
   C. Disseminated intravascular coagulation
   D. Pancreatitis
   E. Transfusion
   F. Uremia
   G. High altitude
   H. Rapid evacuation of pneumothorax and hydrothorax

formation. Finally, increased negative interstitial pressure secondary to rapid removal by suction of large pleural effusions or pneumothoraces may be followed by pulmonary edema.

Altered permeability is the prototype of noncardiogenic pulmonary edema. Different pathophysiologic mechanisms have been proposed for the alveolar-capillary injury. These mechanisms include microemboli, platelets, leukocytes, disseminated intravascular coagulation, infectious agents or their products, inhaled and circulating toxins, vasoactive substances (histamine, serotonin, kinins), immunologic reactions, complement, oxygen, and the central nervous system. Because of the many clinical conditions associated with the adult respiratory distress syndrome, some or all of these mechanisms may be operative.

Differences between the hydrostatic and permeability types of pulmonary edema can be seen in Figure 5.9. Greater increases in lymphatic flow and fluid and protein movement into the lung are found for similar increases in hydrostatic pressures in permeability types of edema as compared to

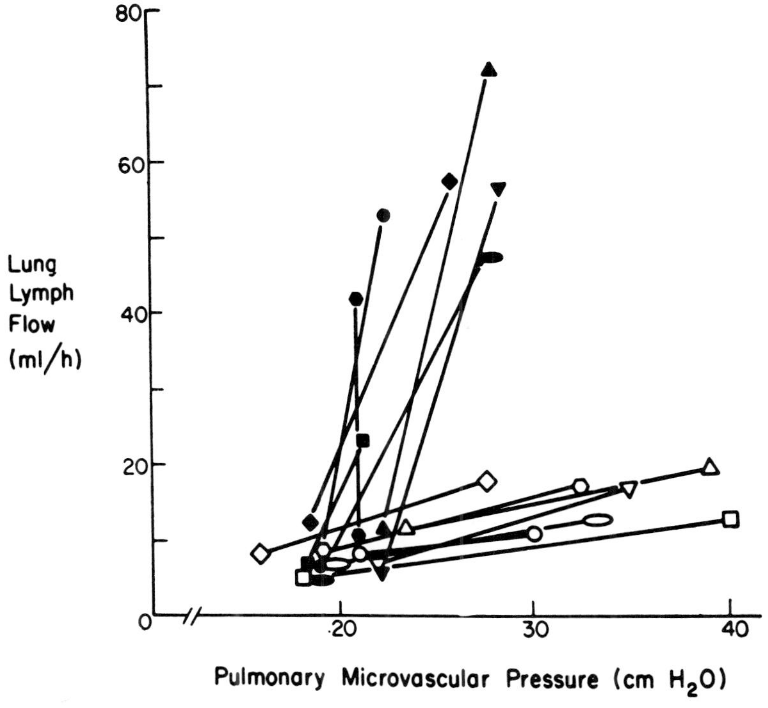

Figure 5.9. Comparison of lymph flow as a function of pulmonary microvascular hydrostatic pressure in sheep before and after increases in left atrial pressure *(open symbol)* and increased permeability induced by *Pseudomonas* bacteremia *(closed symbol)*. For any increase in pulmonary hydrostatic pressure, lymph flow increases are much greater for permeability as opposed to hydrostatic manipulations. Reproduced from Brigham, 1974 (27) with permission.

hydrostatic (increased pulmonary capillary pressure) forms of pulmonary edema (27).

Recently, pulmonary edema fluid analysis has proved helpful in identifying the different types of pulmonary edema. Only patients with severe forms of pulmonary edema produce pulmonary edema fluid. Patients with cardiogenic pulmonary edema have high hydrostatic pressures. The microvascular membrane remains intact and the pulmonary edema is a "transudate." The colloid osmotic pressure or total protein concentration ratio of pulmonary edema fluid to serum in these patients is typically low. Noncardiogenic pulmonary edema secondary to altered permeability is related to an abnormal microvascular membrane, and the pulmonary edema fluid to serum protein ratio approaches one.

On examination of patients with pure cardiac and noncardiac etiologies of pulmonary edema, there is still an overlap of edema fluid to serum protein ratios (Figure 5.10) (28). No patient with a noncardiac etiology had an edema fluid to serum total protein ratio less than 0.5, however, and no patient with a cardiac etiology had a protein ratio greater than 0.7. Therefore, patients with edema fluid to serum total protein ratios less than 0.5 can be categorized as cardiogenic pulmonary edema (CPE) cases and those patients with ratios greater than 0.7 can be classified as noncardiogenic pulmonary edema (NCPE) cases (28). We have designated those patients with ratios between 0.5 and 0.7 as cases of intermediate pulmonary edema. Differentiation of cardiac and noncardiac etiologies of pulmonary edema in these patients can be determined by the edema fluid to serum globulin ratio; patients with noncardiac etiologies have ratios greater than 0.52, whereas patients with cardiac etiologies have ratios less than or equal to 0.52 (28). Based on these edema fluid to serum ratios, one can determine the type of pulmonary edema and look for a more specific etiology. In addition, patients with NCPE typically require pulmonary artery catheterization. If one can demonstrate by fluid analyses that NCPE is present, catheterization need not wait for a response to therapy which most likely will not occur.

It is important to realize that patients may have more than one etiology for pulmonary edema formation. Despite the fact that permeability types of pulmonary edema are defined by a normal hydrostatic pressure, some patients may have a permeability defect (secondary to sepsis, pneumonia, etc.) but may also have increased hydrostatic pressure secondary to volume overload or myocardial dysfunction (29).

The basic goal in ARDS is to provide oxygen delivery to vital organs and supportive care until the pathologic process has abated and/or the lungs have begun to heal. Continuous positive airway pressure (CPAP) by facemasks can occasionally be used but tracheal intubation is usually required to administer high concentrations of oxygen and positive end-expiratory pressure (PEEP). Patients are typically hyperventilating, but ventilatory as-

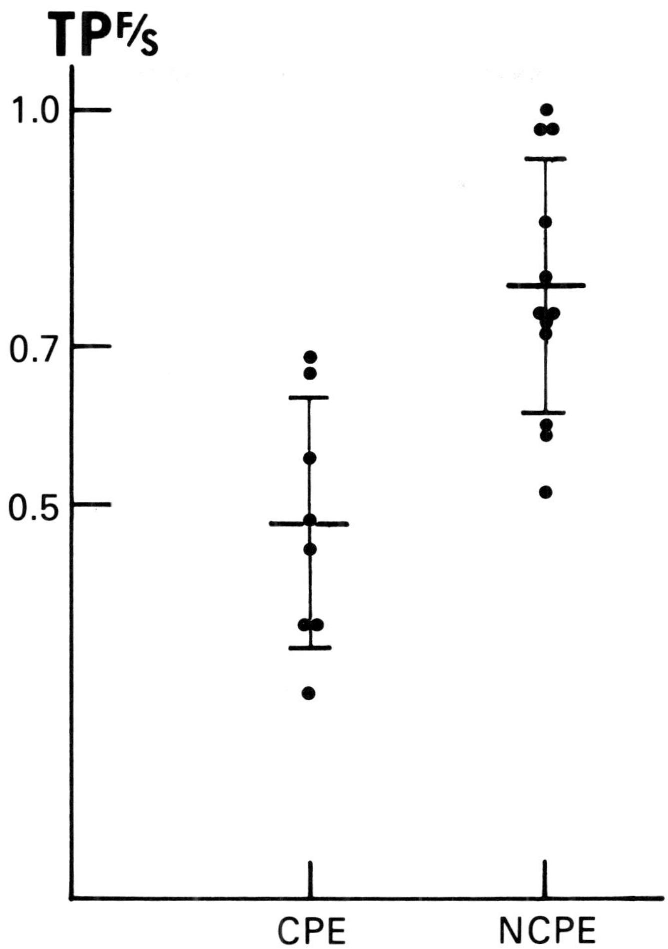

Figure 5.10. Edema fluid (F) to serum (S) total protein (TP) ratios in patients with cardiac (CPE) and noncardiac (NCPE) pulmonary edema. Only patients with CPE have ratios less than 0.5 whereas only NCPE patients have ratios greater than 0.7. Unfortunately even in these classical patients with CPE and NCPE there is still an overlap in the permeability defects.

sistance may be required secondary to the reduced lung compliance and increased work of breathing. Volume-cycled or time-cycled respirators must be used in ARDS because the decreased lung compliance causes high pressures which pressure-cycled ventilators can not overcome if the required tidal volumes are to be delivered. The dilemma of therapy in ARDS is that the high concentrations of inspired oxygen necessary to overcome the hypoxemia due to right to left intrapulmonary shunting are toxic to the lung and can produce a syndrome indistinguishable from the primary process. The application of PEEP, by placing the expiratory tubing of the ventilator under a measured depth of water, has been shown to result in a higher pO_2 at a given FIO_2. This helps avoid oxygen toxicity by allowing oxygenation of tissues at a lower FIO_2. PEEP acts by reinflating collapsed lung units and redistributing fluid in partially air-filled alveoli so that the fluid is around the periphery of the alveoli, decreasing the barrier to diffusion. It has been proposed by some that PEEP also may act by "pushing" water back into pulmonary capillaries, and therefore, decrease lung water. This effect has not been demonstrated experimentally, however, and is not widely accepted.

PEEP is not without adverse effects. Recognized complications are barotrauma (pneumothorax, pneumomediastinum, and subcutaneous emphysema) and decreased cardiac output. Cardiac output is believed to decrease secondary to decreased venous return to the right heart, increased pulmonary vascular resistance, or changes in the pericardium, ventricular septum or the left ventricular cavity (30). Because of this decrease in cardiac output with increasing PEEP, a point of diminishing return can be reached; increasing PEEP with an increase in pO_2 can cause a significant decrease in cardiac output and impaired oxygen delivery. Therefore, whenever more than minimal amounts of PEEP are used (greater than 5 to 10 cm H_2O), pulmonary artery catheterization should be performed. Measurements of cardiac output and of arterial and mixed venous blood gases, and calculations of oxygen delivery, arterial-mixed venous oxygen content differences, and pulmonary shunt can be performed.

The definition of "best PEEP" is controversial (31, 32). Some physicians consider PEEP optimal when oxygen delivery is highest and any further increase in PEEP decreases oxygen delivery (31). Others have used the PEEP which decreases the pulmonary shunt to less than 15% as the optimal PEEP (32). We have used oxygen delivery as a basis for best PEEP and have only used that amount of PEEP which will enable us to decrease the FIO_2 to presumably nontoxic concentrations (FIO_2 = 0.4 - 0.5).

Careful attention must be given to the fluid balance of patients with ARDS. As noted previously, permeability defects cause an increase in the movement of water and protein into the lung. This has been demonstrated in the experimental animal (See Figure 5.9) (27) and in actual patients (Figure 5.11) (33). Therefore, in order to alter the lung water distribution for the maximum benefit of these patients, the lowest hydrostatic pressure (PWP) compatible with good tissue perfusion should be maintained. Therapy requires water and sodium restriction and usually potent diuretics such as furosemide. Because PEEP can decrease venous return and cardiac output, PWP can usually not be decreased to too low a level. A PWP of 5-10 mm Hg is, therefore, a realistic target. If the cardiac output does decrease with PEEP, vasopressor agents or fluid infusions can reverse the decreased output. Because of the permeability defect, vasopressor therapy may be preferred to

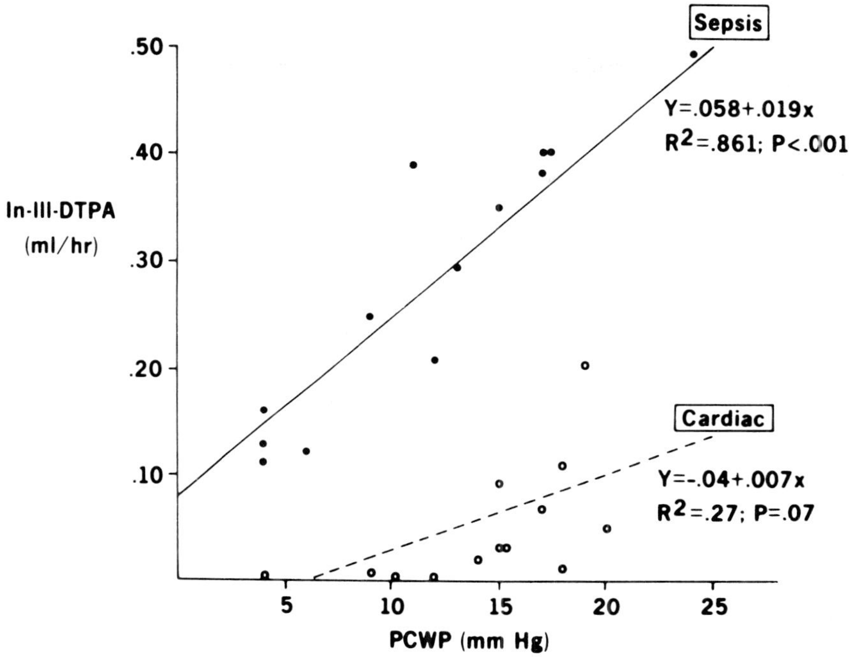

Figure 5.11. Clearance of ^{111}In-labeled diethylene triamine pentaacetic acid (DTPA) as related to pulmonary artery wedge pressure (PCWP). For any change in PCWP, both the slope ($P < 0.005$) and the intercept ($P < 0.01$) were greater in patients with noncardiac edema when compared to patients with cardiac edema. This is similar to the previously noted findings in the animal model noted in Figure 5.9. Reproduced from Sibbald et al., 1981 (32) with permission.

fluid resuscitation. This use of vasopressor agents before obtaining an optimal left ventricular filling pressure is different than other hypoperfusion states.

If fluid therapy is given to patients with ARDS, the question of using crystalloid or colloid (albumin, plasma, dextran) solutions arises. Colloids might be useful if they could maintain or increase intravascular colloid osmotic pressure and decrease fluid movement from pulmonary capillaries. Unfortunately, the capillary endothelium is permeable to even large proteins in ARDS and the colloids may leak into the lung and draw even more fluid with them. We have, therefore, tried to avoid colloids in ARDS, especially if a permeability defect can be determined by pulmonary edema fluid analyses. Others, however, have used colloids successfully even in ARDS. In view of the permeability defect in ARDS, one must always observe for possible worsening of the parameters of oxygenation whenever any type of fluid is given.

Because the lung reacts in the same fashion to many different types of insults (see Table 5.2) and we have not as yet elucidated the pathophysiologic mechanisms of disease for all the various etiologies of ARDS, therapy remains supportive and rather nonspecific. Recent evidence of granulocyte aggregation in the pulmonary microvasculature and complement system activation in association with ARDS have suggested a possible role for the use of corticosteroids in ARDS (34). In fact, Sibbald and colleagues have demonstrated that corticosteroids can decrease permeability once alterations have occurred (35). There is, however, no evidence that steroids favorably affect the outcome of ARDS in humans. A prospective study is currently in progress.

The present patient developed noncardiogenic pulmonary edema and the adult respiratory distress syndrome after treatment for acute upper gastrointestinal bleeding. The pulmonary edema was considered to be noncardiogenic because of the edema fluid to serum colloid osmotic pressure ratio that was 75% and the normal pulmonary artery wedge pressure. The pulmonary edema was initially thought to be secondary to several possible etiologies, as is often the case. These included shock, volume overload secondary to blood transfusions and salt solutions, embolization secondary to blood products or the gelfoam used for the clotting procedure, and aspiration (which is usually very difficult to rule out with absolute certainty). The pulmonary artery catheter was placed to evaluate the exact PWP and to monitor cardiopulmonary variables which would optimize PEEP therapy. The normal PWP and cardiac index made volume overload and cardiac dysfunction unlikely causes of the pulmonary edema. Further definition of the etiology was impossible, but this had no effect on the therapeutic management.

The patient initially had a good cardiac index but because of the increased heart rate had a low SVI and LVSW (profile #1). The pO_2 of 72 mm Hg was acceptable, but the toxic-inspired oxygen concentration of 0.8 indicated a need for more PEEP to increase compliance and enable a decrease in FIO_2. Despite the acceptable oxygen transport, the pvO_2 was decreased and the $avDO_2$ and O_2 utilization ratio were increased. This may have been secondary to the patient's increased metabolic requirements as reflected by the tachycardia, tachypnea, and increased oxygen consumption.

PEEP levels are typically increased by 3- to 5-cm H_2O increments. When PEEP was increased to 10 cm H_2O (profile #2) there was little change in cardiac parameters, and the pO_2 increased. This enabled the physicians to decrease the FIO_2 to 0.7. At this time the pvO_2 increased slightly and the $avDO_2$ decreased slightly. Contractility may have decreased as the CI remained the same with a higher PWP. One must remember, however, that left ventricular pressures may not reflect left ventricular volume in these patients (36) and many investigators have not seen a decrease in contractility with PEEP (37).

When PEEP was increased to 15 cm H_2O, cardiac function deteriorated—BP, CI, SVI, and LVSW decreased. Because of this, oxygen transport also decreased. The decrease in cardiac output was not surprising as cardiac output usually decreases at PEEP levels of 10-15 cm H_2O (37). Dopamine was started because of the decrease in cardiac output and oxygen transport and because the systolic blood pressure decreased to levels lower than 90 mm Hg. Mixed venous oxygen tension did not decrease, despite the decreased oxygen delivery. This is consistent with previous reports in patients with ARDS in whom decreasing oxygen delivery led to similar decreases in oxygen consumption but variable changes in pvO_2 (38). In fact, the pvO_2 had no consistent relation to cardiac output or oxygen delivery (38). By using dopamine, the cardiac output was increased to 7.2 liters/min, CI to 4.2 liters/min/m^2 SVI to 31.4 ml/min/m^2, LVSW to 39 grams·m/m^2, and oxygen transport to 1009 ml O_2/min. PEEP was gradually increased to 20 cm H_2O because the pO_2 was still only 64 mm Hg on an FIO_2 of 0.7 and 15 cm H_2O of PEEP. At this level of PEEP, cardiac function was maintained and the pO_2 increased to 102 mm Hg (profile #4). At this time the pvO_2 increased and the oxygen utilization ratio decreased further. The oxygen transport remained decreased from baseline and previous levels most likely because of the minimal increase in oxygen saturation (despite large changes in pO_2), the minimal decrease in cardiac output, and the decrease in hemoglobin. Subsequent to this, the FIO_2 was decreased to 0.5 and the pO_2 was 70 mm Hg. Because the patient was now on dopamine to maintain cardiac output and was on high levels of PEEP to maintain a pO_2 of 70 mm Hg on 0.5 FIO_2, PEEP therapy was maintained at 20 cm H_2O. Further increases in PEEP were not used, despite an intrapulmonary shunt that was greater than 30% and the fact that an FIO_2 of 0.5 was still required. Other physicians may have increased PEEP further to decrease the shunt or the inspired oxygen concentration.

The present patient's cardiopulmonary alterations during treatment with PEEP were representative of the many changes that occur in patients with ARDS. PEEP increased compliance and pO_2 and enabled a decrease in the FIO_2; pvO_2 increased and $avDO_2$ decreased. As PEEP was increased, the cardiac output fell and dopamine was required. In contrast to the original description of optimal PEEP by Suter (31), many patients will not have increases in measured compliance, despite increasing levels of PEEP. In addition, PEEP will often decrease cardiac output and oxygen transport before adequate oxygenation on nontoxic inspired oxygen concentrations is obtained. Under these circumstances, vasopressors such as dopamine are required to increase cardiac output and oxygen transport so that PEEP can be increased further.

PATIENT 7: MULTIPLE TRAUMA/Joseph M. Civetta

A 39-year-old white male pedestrian was hit by an automobile at 11:00 p.m. Fire-Rescue responded to the emergency call within 5 minutes. The patient was profoundly hypotensive and had obvious fractures. He was placed in the Military Anti-Shock Trousers which were inflated to 100 mm Hg. Intravenous fluids were administered at the scene; however, he remained hypotensive.

On arrival in the Emergency Room, his blood pressure was 60 mm Hg by palpation and initial assessment of his injuries included bilateral open tibia and fibula fractures, right radial fracture, fractures of both pelvic rami, and multiple lacerations of the head and face. Abdominal exam revealed diffuse tenderness and an open peritoneal lavage was performed returning grossly bloody fluid. He was immediately transported to the Operating Room. A laparotomy was performed revealing a major liver laceration and a partially avulsed gall bladder. It was noted that the patient had a previous splenectomy. The lacerations of the head and neck were repaired. The open fractures were cleansed and debrided. Fasciotomies were necessary because of severe muscle swelling in both legs. The operative procedure consumed 6 hours, and 20 units of blood were required to maintain resuscitation. Twenty-one liters of Ringer's Lactate, 6 units of fresh frozen plasma, and 12 platelet transfusions were also administered.

On admission to the Intensive Care Unit a pulmonary artery catheter was placed. At this time the PWP was 8 mm Hg and the cardiac output was 8 liters/min. Determination of arterial and mixed venous blood gases showed arterial pO_2 of 86 mm Hg ($FIO_2 = 0.45$) and a mixed venous saturation of 49%; $avDO_2$ was 7 ml/dl and intrapulmonary shunt (Qs/Qt) was 14%. During the ensuing 12 hours, 3 units of whole blood and 4 liters of crystalloid solution were required to maintain hemoglobin, cardiac output and urinary output. Repetitive sampling of arterial oxygen tension showed diminution requiring an increase in positive end-expiratory pressure. At 15 cm H_2O of PEEP, cardiac output was 7.2 liters/min, wedge pressure was 11 mm Hg, and intrapulmonary shunt again was 15%. Approximately 2 hours later cardiac output had fallen to 5.9 liters/min, however, and dopamine 200 μg/min was initiated. After this intervention, cardiac output increased to 10.8 liters/min and the wedge pressure decreased to 8 mm Hg. Blood gases at this time showed an arterial pO_2 of 59 mm Hg, mixed venous saturation of 53%, and an arterial venous oxygen content difference of 7.3 ml/dl. Intrapulmonary shunt was 10%. During the next 24 hours, arterial blood gases continued to improve after administration of whole blood to raise his hemoglobin to 12.7 grams/dl. Because of increased systolic blood pressure, dopamine was discontinued; however, cardiac output fell to 5.9 liters/min and an infusion of dobutamine (400 μg/min) was started. This produced an increase in cardiac output to 10.5 liters/min without increasing systolic blood pressure. Mixed venous saturation increased to 65% and PEEP could be progressively increased to improve arterial oxygenation to 134 mm Hg. At this time, the shunt was 8.2%. This required incremental application of PEEP to 28 cm H_2O.

In the third 24-hour period, his cardiorespiratory situation improved and PEEP was progressively weaned to 18 cm H_2O. Dobutamine could be decreased to 200 μg/min and the cardiac output was 10.4 liters/min; arterial pO_2 was 124 mm Hg, $avDO_2$ was 6.3 ml/dl, and shunt was 11%.

On the fourth ICU day, whereas PEEP was maintained at 18 cm H_2O, dobutamine was discontinued with cardiac output remaining between 8.4 and

10.5 liters/min on numerous determinations. A positive fluid balance of approximately 2.5 liters of crystalloid was necessary on each of the first 3 days. Over the next 24 hours it was possible to wean the PEEP progressively from 18 to 12 cm H_2O with essentially no change in cardiovascular or respiratory function. Spontaneous diuresis occurred during the next 48 hours; however, blood gases deteriorated with an increase in intrapulmonary shunt to 31%. PEEP was again incrementally added until 24 cm H_2O was reached. At this point, intrapulmonary shunt decreased to 12.9%, cardiac output without inotropic support was 13.3 liters/min, arterial pO_2 was 106 mm Hg, mixed venous saturation 65%, and $avDO_2$ was 5.3 ml/dl. Progressive weaning was then attempted over the next 48 hours with intermittent success. Intrapulmonary shunt was maintained between 10% and 15% until PEEP levels had been reduced to 16 cm H_2O. At this time shunt increased to 24% requiring an increase in positive end-expiratory pressure. Cardiac output was maintained between 10 and 12 liters/min without inotropic support. On the 10th intensive care day, intrapulmonary shunt again increased to 25% and PEEP was raised from 24 to 26 cm H_2O. This reduced shunt to 15%. Cardiac output ranged from 9.4 to 10.5 liters/min. On the 12th intensive care day, spiking temperatures were noted to 103° F. Sequential blood cultures, sputum cultures, and urine cultures revealed no pathogens. The chest x-ray showed a diffuse interstitial infiltrate without evidence of pneumonia. Sputum gram stain showed rare gram-negative rods without white blood cells. Examination of the abdomen revealed diffuse abdominal tenderness. Serum amylase was elevated to 193 units. Liver function studies showed a total bilirubin of 2.4 mg/dl with a direct component of 1.2 mg/dl, SGOT of 102 mU/ml, and serum glutamic pyruvic transaminase (SGPT) of 90 mU/ml. Traumatic pancreatitis and/or cholecystitis were suspected. Abdominal CT scan, pipida scan, and abdominal echo examination suggested a mass in the right upper quadrant. The patient was taken to the Operating Room and a cholecystectomy performed for acute acalculous cholecystitis. During this procedure, cardiac output fell to 7.7 liters/min requiring administration of dobutamine, 400 μg/min. Respiratory function remained stable during this period of time. Over the next 48 hours, PEEP could be progressively weaned in increments to 11 cm H_2O. Cardiac output was 11 liters/min, $avDO_2$ was 3.4 ml/dl, and intrapulmonary shunt was 16.9%. Dobutamine was discontinued without a change in cardiac output.

At this point, his cardiac instability and respiratory failure had resolved and the invasive monitoring devices were removed. His further course was one of slow improvement in respiratory function over the next 2 weeks. He was extubated on the 32nd ICU day. No further cardiovascular interventions were necessary during these 2 weeks. Two days after extubation, his condition was considered stable enough for discharge to an intermediate care unit.

Discussion

This patient presented with severe multisystem trauma and developed post-traumatic respiratory insufficiency. Although the exact etiology was uncertain, he had many known antecendents including long bone fractures, acute alcoholism with vomiting and possible aspiration, and blunt chest trauma. He also suffered a prolonged period of shock and required multiple blood transfusions. It has been our experience, however, that these correlate with the severity of the other antecedents and cannot be directly linked to pulmonary insufficiency. His decreased cardiac output was not always associated with the level of ventilatory support and suggested direct myocardial contusion. No changes were noted in his electrocardiograms, although creatine phosphokinase isoenzymes were slightly elevated. Although the volume of crystalloid infusion may be considered to be large in absolute numbers, it is proportional to the severity of the soft tissue injuries and the magnitude of blood loss. It is interesting to note that the deterioration in respiratory function in association with the development of intra-abdominal sepsis occurred during a period of spontaneous diuresis and that further respiratory support in the second postoperative period could again reverse this change. Because of simultaneous recurring changes in both cardiac and respiratory function, invasive monitoring was necessary not only to define the abnormalities of cardiovascular function but also to allow discrimination between respiratory and cardiac function in terms of their independent effects on arterial oxygen tension. The lowest arterial oxygen tensions were not accompanied by the largest deteriorations in respiratory function as estimated by intrapulmonary shunt, but rather correlated with the lowest mixed venous oxygen tensions. At that point, therapy was directed to improve oxygen delivery both by administration of additional red cell mass as well as the resultant effects upon increasing ventricular filling pressures. Finally, inotropic agents were necessary to maintain cardiovascular function during the highest levels of end-expiratory pressure in the immediate postoperative course, and secondarily, to support the depressed myocardial function associated with the intra-abdominal sepsis. The complete information afforded by invasive monitoring in all three areas: pressure, flow, and mixed venous sampling, perhaps, can be underscored in terms of the tenacity of approach necessary to achieve this end: 5 pulmonary artery catheters were required (by our 72-hour duration protocol) and 68 cardiorespiratory profiles performed during this period.

PATIENT 8: PREOPERATIVE EVALUATION FOR SURGERY/Bradley H. Ruben

A 70-year-old woman was scheduled for an elective abdominal-perineal resection for carcinoma of the sigmoid colon. The patient had hypertension for 15 years which was well controlled with a diuretic and an oral antihypertensive agent. The patient led a sedentary life, and gave no history of physical limitations in her daily routine. Physical examination revealed an obese, elderly woman, with a blood pressure of 160/100 mm Hg. The preoperative chest x-ray showed clear lung fields but the electrocardiogram revealed nonspecific ST-T wave changes. The patient was hospitalized for several days preoperatively. Her blood pressure was noted to range from 145 to 185 mm Hg systolic and 95 to 115 mm Hg diastolic. The patient was brought to the intensive care

Profile Chart 5.5. Cardiopulmonary profile of elderly patient preoperatively

Enter:	**Date/time:** # 1	# 2
Cardiac output (CO)	4.0	5.2
Systolic blood pressure (SBP)	160	150
Diastolic blood pressure (DBP)	100	90
Mean arterial pressure (MAP)	120	110
Heart rate (HR)	85	70
Mean pulmonary artery pressure (MPAP)	26	24
Pulmonary artery wedge pressure (PWP)	15	10
Central venous pressure (CVP)	8	6
Body surface area (BSA)	2.1	2.1
Data:		
Stroke volume (SV)	47.1	74.3
Cardiac index (CI)	1.9	2.5
Stroke index (SI)	22.4	35.4
Right ventricular stroke work (RVSW)	5	9
RVSW/CVP ratio	0.63	1.5
Left ventricular stroke work (LVSW)	32	48
LVSW/PWP ratio	2.13	4.8
Systemic vascular resistance (SVR)	2237	1598
Pulmonary vascular resistance (PVR)	220	215
Enter:		
Hemoglobin (Hgb)	14	14
FIO_2	0.21	0.21
$PaCO_2$	40	40
PaO_2	68	70
SaO_2	0.94	0.95
$P\bar{v}O_2$	36	40
$S\bar{v}O_2$	0.65	0.70
DATA:		
Capillary O_2 content (CcO_2)	19.3	19.3
Mixed venous O_2 content ($C\bar{v}O_2$)	12.5	13.4
Arterial O_2 content (CaO_2)	18.1	18.3
Arteriovenous O_2 content difference ($avDO_2$)	5.6	4.9
O_2 delivery	724	952
O_2 consumption (VO_2)	224	255
O_2 utilization ratio	0.31	0.27
Intrapulmonary shunt (Qs/Qt)	0.18	0.17
PaO_2/FIO_2	324	333
Vasopressors or vasodilators (μ/k/m)		

unit prior to her scheduled operation for placement of a pulmonary artery catheter. The cardiopulmonary data obtained can be seen in Profile Chart 5.5, profile #1. The patient's operation was cancelled and she was digitalized over the next 24 hours. The cardiopulmonary profile on the next day is noted in Profile Chart 5.5, profile #2. She was taken to the operating room for her surgical procedure. The 3½-hour surgical procedure was uneventful. She required 2 units of whole blood and 4.5 liters of crystalloid solution in the operating room. Upon return to the ICU, the patient was found to have a temperature of 95° F and a blood pressure of 215/130 mm Hg. The cardiac output was 4.5 liters/min; systemic vascular resistance (SVR), 2808 dyne·sec·cm^{-5}; the CVP, 10 mm Hg; PWP, 14 mm Hg; and avDO$_2$, 6 ml/dl. The patient was given medication for pain and placed on a warming blanket, and nitroprusside was used to lower her mean arterial pressure between 110 and 120 mm Hg. After the patient was warmed and the mean arterial pressure was 120 mm Hg, the cardiac output increased to 6 liters/min and the SVR was 1600 dyne·sec·cm^{-5}. The remainder of her ICU stay was uneventful. She was weaned from the nitroprusside and was discharged to the floor 24 hours postoperatively.

Discussion

It is estimated that approximately 35 million people (1 out of 6) in the United States have hypertension. Less than half of these individuals have been diagnosed as having hypertension and less than 20% of those diagnosed have received appropriate therapy. The anesthesiologist is concerned with the severity of hypertension, its duration and the degree of impairment to the target organs—the brain, kidney, and heart. The patient with longstanding hypertension often has coronary artery disease and/or left ventricular hypertrophy which may not only diminish the oxygen supply to the heart but may also increase oxygen requirements. Patients with severe hypertension are at risk for the development of myocardial ischemia or infarction during or after surgery (39). Patients who are taking medication which controls their hypertension have a lesser incidence of these complications (39). In addition, patients with a history of hypertension tend to have blood pressure lability intraoperatively. If these intraoperative blood pressure swings are treated and avoided, there are decreased cardiovascular complications postoperatively (40). Table 5.3 notes the major disorders which increase the anesthetic risk for surgery.

In addition to the problem of hypertension, this patient was also elderly. The proportion of people in the United States above 65 years of age is estimated to be approximately 11%. The proportion of elderly patients is even higher in the hospital population, ranging between 12% and 35% (41). Even in the absence of associated diseases, postoperative mortality is considerably higher in elderly patients when compared to young adults. Above the age of 80, mortality of elective surgery may be as high as 14%, whereas that of emergency surgery may reach 44% (41). In the young and in the aged,

Table 5.3. Disorders that increase anesthetic risk

I. Cardiovascular
  A. Primary myocardial problems (in association with a left ventricular ejection fraction < 40%)
  B. Segmental wall motion abnormalities
  C. Ventricular aneurysm
  D. Global dysfunction

II. Fixed cardiac output
  A. Aortic stenosis
  B. Mitral stenosis
  C. Pacemaker-dependent arrhythmias
  D. Constrictive pericarditis or cardiac tamponade
  E. Massive pulmonary embolism

III. Ischemic heart disease
  A. Previous myocardial infarction
  B. Recent myocardial infarction
  C. Unstable angina
  D. Narrowing of left main coronary artery

IV. Congenital heart disease
  A. Eisenmenger's syndrome
  B. Left to right shunts with pulmonary hypertension
  C. Other severe mechanical defects

V. Conduction defects or arrhythmias
  A. Sinoatrial disease
  B. Bifascicular block
  C. High-grade atrioventricular block
  D. Prolonged QT-interval syndrome

VI. Serious pulmonary disease
  A. Hypoventilation
  B. Right-to-left intrapulmonary shunt
  C. Impaired diffusing capacity
  D. Ventilation/perfusion inequality

VII. Hypovolemia
  A. Blood loss
  B. Third-space sequestration of fluid
  C. Dehydration

VIII. Endocrine dysfunction
  A. Adrenal insufficiency
  B. Thyroid dysfunction
  C. Brittle insulin-dependent diabetes

IX. Nervous system disorders
  A. Advanced peripheral neuropathy
  B. Cerebrovascular disease
  C. Myasthenia gravis

X. Serious renal or hepatic impairment

Originally published in Canadian Medical Association Journal, October 6, 1979.

postoperative mortality is dramatically increased by the presence of associated diseases, especially acute illnesses (41). According to Powers (42), the incidence of cardiovascular disease is 6% in the fifth decade, 23% in the sixth decade, 45% in the seventh decade, and 100% in the eighth decade. Surgical mortality is influenced considerably by the presence of cardiovascular disease. There is a higher surgical mortality in patients with cardiovascular disease than in those patients without heart disease. Patients with pre-existing cardiovascular and pulmonary disease before surgery have an increased likelihood for those complications to worsen postoperatively, especially when there is preoperative hypertension or intraoperative hypotension, or in thoracic or upper abdominal operations or operations lasting more than 3 hours (39, 40).

Del Guercio and Cohn (43) studied 148 consecutive patients over the age of 65 years by placing a pulmonary artery catheter in these patients preoperatively. All patients had been cleared for surgery by standard medical assessment. Only 13.5% of these patients had normal measured hemodynamic, respiratory, and oxygen transport functions. Mild physiologic abnormalities that did not require a delay in surgery, or more severe abnormalities that were indications of high operative risk were found in 63.5% of their patients. Advanced and uncorrectable functional defects were found in the remaining 23% and this made them unacceptable risks for major surgery under general anesthesia. Del Guercio concluded that invasive preoperative assessment of patients over 65 years of age can disclose a high percentage of serious physiologic abnormalities which may require a delay or cancellation of a proposed operation in many patients.

Intraoperative volume replacement and volume loss are traditionally estimated by the anesthesiologist by means that are at best indirect. Blood loss is estimated by "eye-balling" the surgical field and drapes, the number of surgical sponges and the saturation of these sponges by blood. At best, this is very subjective, and the possibility of error is more pronounced with greater blood loss. Adequacy of blood volume has traditionally been estimated by adequacy of urine volume and by CVP. As noted elsewhere in this book, the CVP may not be a good indicator of volume status and PWP monitoring may be more indicative of left atrial filling pressure and volume requirements. Whether preoperative, operative, or postoperative hemodynamic monitoring will improve the survival of various groups of patients such as the elderly remains to be determined. Invasive monitoring, however, can certainly identify cardiopulmonary abnormalities that may not be apparent by standard noninvasive medical assessment. These patients may benefit from physiologic "fine tuning" before or during their operative procedures.

A pulmonary artery catheter was inserted in this patient preoperatively because of the patient's age, the presence of mild but uncontrolled hypertension, and the potential of a prolonged operative procedure with large fluid volume loss. The patient demonstrated a hypodynamic pattern with a low cardiac index and high systemic vascular resistance. Early heart failure may have been present with the increased hydrostatic filling pressures. Inadequate oxygen delivery was manifested by a low pvO_2 and widened arteriovenous oxygen difference. Her hypertension had been apparently controlled before hospitalization but her hypertension became mildly elevated prior to surgery. This increase in afterload probably caused her left ventricle to fail. After digitalization, improvement in the hemodynamic parameters was noted and she had an uneventful intraoperative course. Postoperatively, the patient was hypertensive. This was most likely secondary to her hypothermia and emergence from anesthesia with concomitant pain perception. The pulmonary artery catheter was in place, and the pulmonary artery wedge pressure was normal. Inadequate oxygen delivery was present as evidenced by the widened $avDO_2$. Flow was improved by simple vasodilation. The availability of the pulmonary artery catheter at this time enabled the physicians to treat the patient with the appropriate therapy based on physiologic data rather than clinical suspicions. There was no need for fluid resuscitation or inotropic support.

PATIENT 9: CARDIAC SURGERY/Bradley H. Ruben

A 61-year-old man was scheduled for a triple coronary artery bypass graft. He had a 7-year history of stable angina controlled on propranolol 20 mg four times a day and occasional sublingual nitroglycerin. He was recently admitted to the hospital for an episode of prolonged chest pain which was associated with marked ischemic changes on his electrocardiogram. An acute myocardial infarction was ruled out by serial electrocardiograms and cardiac enzymes. While in the intensive care unit, the patient had several prolonged episodes of chest pain while on an intravenous nitroglycerin drip and propranolol 60 mg every 6 hours. Cardiac catheterization was performed and revealed: heart rate, 55 beats/min; blood pressure, 110/65 mm Hg; cardiac output, 5.5 liters/min; systemic vascular resistance, 1164 dynes·sec·cm^{-5}; $avDO_2$, 4.7 ml/dl; stroke volume, 100 ml/beat; ejection fraction, 87%; left ventricular end-diastolic pressure, 19 mm Hg at rest and 28 mm Hg postangiography; and right ventricular end-diastolic pressure, 7 mm Hg. No valvular abnormalities were noted. The left ventricle demonstrated hypokinesis of the inferior wall. The right coronary artery had an 80% obstruction near its origin. The left anterior descending artery revealed an elongated lesion near the first diagonal branch, estimated as a 90% obstruction of the vessel's lumen. The circumflex artery had a 75% occlusion proximal to the obtuse marginal branch. Arterial oxygenation was normal.

The patient arrived in the operating room after receiving morphine sulfate and scopolamine intramuscularly and diazepam and propranolol orally as preoperative medications. Because of the dyskinetic inferior myocardial wall segment and the disparity between the right atrial pressure and the left atrial pressure, a pulmonary artery catheter was inserted via the right internal jugular vein. A radial artery catheter was also inserted for continuous blood pressure monitoring. Lead II and lead V_5 were continuously monitored for rhythm and evidence of ST-T wave changes. The pulmonary artery catheter revealed the following preoperative data: CVP, 5 mm Hg; PWP, 12 mm Hg; and cardiac output, 5 liters/min. Induction of anesthesia was started by a slow infusion of fentanyl with an additional 10 mg of diazepam, intravenously. After the appropriate amount of fentanyl was infused, pancuronium was also infused to facilitate intubation. During this period, respirations were controlled by face mask with 100% oxygen. Heart rate remained between 55 and 65 beats/min while the blood pressure and PWP remained at preinduction levels. Concurrent with placement of the endotracheal tube, the patient's heart rate rose to 100 beats/min and the systolic blood pressure rose to 140 mm Hg. The patient was now anesthetized. If myocardial ischemia occurred, the patient was unable to express the sensation of chest pain. At this time, the rate-pressure product was greater than 12,000 which is associated with increased myocardial oxygen demands (44). The rapid addition of further anesthesia was therefore indicated to abate the increased sympathetic response to tracheal stimulation. Consequently, halothane, an inhalational anesthetic, was added in small concentrations. This produced a decrease in the heart rate to 80 beats/min and a fall in the blood pressure to 100/50 mm Hg. At this time, the development of ST-T wave changes was noted in lead V_5. Because halothane can decrease preload by peripheral vasodilation and decrease myocardial contractility directly, a rapid means to assess myocardial function was required. The PWP at this time was 20 mm Hg. In the face of ischemic ECG changes and a decrease in the coronary perfusion pressure (diastolic blood pressure minus left ventricular end-diastolic pressure), improvement in myocardial contractility to increase oxygen delivery was obtained by the intravenous titration of calcium chloride. This counteracted the myocardial depressant effects of the halothane. The blood pressure then increased to 120/70 mm Hg and at the same time the PWP decreased to 15 mm Hg. If the PWP had not been known, additional fluid may have been given to increase the preload and blood pressure. In this case, fluid therapy would have been inappropriate and may have led to the development of pulmonary edema. The immediate postinduction period is very critical in that rapid changes in hemodynamic parameters require rapid assessment and appropriate interventions. Because rapid interventions are often required to prevent disastrous complications, the luxury of performing cardiac output determinations is not always possible.

After adequate anesthesia, the surgical incision and sternotomy caused no change in the heart rate, blood pressure, or PWP. During 2 hours of cardiopulmonary bypass, three aorto-coronary venous grafts were placed. While coming off bypass the blood pressure was well maintained by keeping the PWP at 15 mm Hg with fluid from the cardiopulmonary bypass pump. Once off bypass, the blood pressure and PWP began to decrease slowly. Because the hematocrit was only 28%, red blood cells were infused to maintain the PWP at 15 mm Hg which also maintained the systolic blood pressure (SBP) at 110 mm Hg. While closing the sternum, the blood pressure dropped despite a PWP of 18 mm Hg. The cardiac output was noted to be 3.8 liters/min at this time. The patient was placed on 5 μg/kg/min of dopamine which increased the cardiac output to 4.8 liters/min with a PWP of 15 mm Hg. The patient was taken to the intensive care unit where he was weaned from the dopamine and extubated the same day. He proceeded to make an uneventful recovery.

Discussion

Anesthesia is an abnormal physiologic state in which most normal physiologic responses are minimized or abated. Anesthesia in the normal individual produces alterations in the homeostatic responses which affect the heart, brain, lungs, and kidneys. The abolition of consciousness itself can alter cardiovascular responses due to changes in central sympathetic and parasympathetic systems. Manipulation of the airway or surgical stimulation during light anesthesia, will elicit profound autonomic responses. Under these circumstances a dramatic increase in catecholamine concentrations and their associated hemodynamic changes including tachycardia, hypertension, arrhythmias, and increased peripheral vascular resistance may occur. Tachycardia decreases coronary blood flow and oxygen supply secondary to a shortened diastolic time, whereas hypertension increases myocardial work and oxygen demand. These physiologic changes may be extremely hazardous to a patient with compromised myocardial perfusion due to coronary atherosclerosis. Myocardial ischemia, ischemic arrhythmias, and/or pump failure may occur very rapidly leading to cardiovascular collapse. The induction of anesthesia, therefore, should be a "straight line" or steady state situation in patients who have myocardial ischemia or heart failure. Anesthesiologists typically consider the determinants of myocardial oxygen supply and demand in performing a smooth induction in the cardiac patient. Minimizing myocardial oxygen demand is obtained by: abating preinduction anxiety, keeping the heart rate normal through induction, giving adequate levels of anesthesia and analgesia and keeping left ventricular filling pressures normal or low. Maximizing myocardial oxygen supply is obtained by: again keeping the heart rate normal, utilizing 100% oxygen during critical periods, keeping the diastolic blood pressure normal, or even slightly elevated to maintain coronary perfusion pressure, and insuring adequate blood carrying capacity for oxygen. The rate-pressure product and the triple index (SBP × HR × PWP) have been used to monitor these patients during surgery. If hypertension or tachycardia occur, the standard methods to treat these abnormalities are also not without adverse consequences. For example, the reduction of afterload by intravenous vasodilators may also decrease the preload and thus decrease cardiac output; the use of beta blockers to treat tachycardia may also decrease myocardial contractility.

All volatile anesthetics currently being used depress myocardial function, cause peripheral vasodilation, and are arrhythmogenic in dose-dependent fashion. Nitrous oxide, used as a second gas along with oxygen for analgesia and amnesia, will depress myocardial contractility in concentrations as low as 40%. When nitrous oxide is used along with a more potent inhalation anesthetic, the concentration of the more potent drug can be reduced in order to obtain the same anesthetic effect. Consequently, the myocardial depressant effects of the volatile anesthetic can be reduced.

With the advent of cardiac surgery, the use of narcotics as primary anesthetics has become popular because they have very little direct effect on myocardial contractility. Large doses of morphine (1-2 mg/kg) given intravenously have little effect on cardiac function directly. Cardiac output may decrease, however, secondary, to an increased venous capacitance and decreased preload. Despite these rather large doses, patients may remain conscious without amnesia and require the use of other drugs such as nitrous oxide, volatile inhalation agents or diazepam. The use of these large doses of morphine may also require prolonged postoperative ventilatory support. The use of the more potent short acting narcotic fentanyl allows larger doses to be used (up to 150 μg/kg) as the primary or sole anesthetic. Unfortunately, fentanyl may also not eliminate awareness or the sympathetic responses to noxious stimuli. Short acting barbiturates such as thiopental, commonly used during the induction of anesthesia, are generally avoided in cardiac anesthesia. If they are used in sufficient dosages to abolish sympathetic responses, they may have a profound cardiovascular depressant effect, especially in those patients who lack cardiovascular reserve.

There is no ideal anesthetic induction or maintenance agent. The primary goals of anesthesia are to prevent awareness and to provide pain relief from noxious stimuli. This is performed while insuring adequate oxygenation, appropriate blood volume replacement, prevention of hypertension and hypotension, and the avoidance of arrhythmias. These goals are met if the operative procedure is performed with optimal cardiac performance and the avoidance of myocardial ischemia. With these goals in mind, anesthesiologists have in their armamentarium various anesthetic techniques to provide not only complete pain relief and lack of awareness but also methods to monitor the patient's physiologic status. These traditional monitoring techniques for surgery include: intra-arterial blood pressure for second-to-second blood pressure monitoring, heart rate and rhythm monitoring by electrocardiography, and monitoring of central venous pressures and of urine output to estimate the volume status. Although these are routinely used for intraoperative monitoring, they are at best indirect tools, with limitations which are even more limited if severe cardiac disease is present. Since the introduction of the pulmonary artery catheter, anesthesiologists have had at their disposal a more sophisticated tool in which to monitor cardiopulmonary performance. As noted elsewhere in this book, cardiac output, systemic and pulmonary vascular resistance, left ventricular volume status, and parameters of oxygenation can be derived rapidly using the pulmonary artery catheter. Anesthesiologists can use these parameters to individualize anesthetic techniques and to adjust their therapies based on the rapid assessment of the physiologic responses to anesthesia.

There are no data to show a decrease in morbidity, mortality, or cost to benefit ratio by using the pulmonary artery catheter intraoperatively. The use of the pulmonary artery catheter as noted in Chapter 3 is not without hazards. Physicians in some institutions in the United States place a pulmonary artery catheter in all patients undergoing coronary artery surgery. In contrast, other physicians believe that routine pulmonary artery catheterization of patients for open heart surgery is hazardous and an added expense. In these institutions the use of the pulmonary artery catheter is reserved for more specific clinical and anatomical abnormalities. A clear indication appears to be those patients who have ejection fractions by cardiac catheterization of less than 40% or those who have two or more ventricular wall segments with dyssynergy. In this patient population, the right atrial pressures as measured by central venous pressures do not predictably correlate with left atrial filling pressures (45). In addition, a recent study showed that intraoperative increases in pulmonary artery wedge pressure are indicative of myocardial ischemia and can be demonstrated to occur even before electrocardiographic changes (46). A second group of patients who would benefit from pulmonary artery monitoring are those patients with valvular heart disease. Patients with fixed cardiac outputs due to their valvular disease may have dramatic changes in cardiac output secondary to decreases in myocardial contractility or alterations in the filling pressures of the heart. In addition, patients with valvular heart disease and pulmonary hypertension have disparate right atrial and left atrial pressures. Further studies will be required to identify the subgroup of patients who benefit from intraoperative hemodynamic monitoring.

The low mortality observed in patients undergoing cardiac surgery is believed to be secondary to the ability to anesthetize patients who have diseased hearts. This has been achieved by the anesthesiologist's understanding of the effects of the various anesthetic choices and techniques upon the myocardium. The advent of the pulmonary artery catheter has certainly increased this understanding.

PATIENT 10: BALLOON OCCLUSION ANGIOGRAPHY/ Charles L. Sprung

A 52-year-old man with an 18-year history of scleroderma was admitted with a 2–3 week history of dysphagia and intermittent, dull, periumbilical pain. The patient had lost 20 pounds in the prior 2 months. Two years before admission, the patient was told he had pulmonary fibrosis. Physical exam revealed an emaciated man with decreased breath sounds, muscle weakness, and sclerodactyly. Gastrointestinal work up showed an esophageal stricture at the gastroesophageal junction and gastric retention secondary to decreased motility. Therapeutic dilatation of the stricture was successful. Peripheral and enteral alimentation was begun but the patient developed a pneumonia which was believed to be secondary to aspiration. Vital signs were normal and on 2 liters of oxygen via nasal cannula the pO_2 was 80 mm Hg. The patient was stable for 3 days, whereupon he developed acute shortness of breath associated with hemoptysis. Physical exam now revealed: pulse, 110 beats/min; BP, 120/80 mm Hg; respirations, 30 breaths/min; and diffuse inspiratory and expiratory rales. Arterial blood gas ($FIO_2 = 1.0$) showed a pH of 7.28, pO_2, 76 mm Hg; and pCO_2, 65 mm Hg. Pulmonary artery catheterization was performed to precisely define the etiology of the respiratory distress and to manage the respiratory failure. The pulmonary artery pressure was 40/22 mm Hg with a pulmonary artery wedge pressure of 15 mm Hg. Because of the strong clinical suspicion of pulmonary emboli, a wedge pulmonary angiogram was performed (Figure 5.12).

Discussion

Although pulmonary angiography is generally considered the "gold standard" for the diagnosis of pulmonary embolism, it can occasionally fail to provide definitive answers. Segmental or subsegmental branches of the pulmonary artery may not be well visualized by standard projections even with selective techniques (47). Bell et al. (48) were the first to describe the use of wedge pulmonary arteriography. Since their original description, other physicians have demonstrated the usefulness of balloon occlusion angiography to supplement and improve standard pulmonary arteriography (47, 49). Wedge arteriography can provide a better visualization of filling defects, small pulmonary vessels and small emboli with a smaller volume of contrast material at lower injection pressures. The diagnosis of pulmonary embolism can be verified or negated in otherwise equivocal cases (47, 49). Special flotation angiography catheters provide for the visualization of a larger pulmonary segment but do not have a thermistor for cardiac output determinations.

The critically ill patient is at a significant risk for the development of pulmonary emboli. Over the last few years, several investigators have advocated the use of bedside balloon occlusion arteriography to diagnose pulmonary emboli in critically ill patients who can not undergo standard pulmonary arteriography (47, 50-53). The procedure is usually performed in patients in whom there is a clinical suspicion of pulmonary embolism, in whom a pulmonary artery catheter has been previously placed for hemodynamic monitoring, and in whom there is an inability or inadvisability to transport the patient for standard pulmonary arteriography (47, 50, 52, 53). After confirmation of appropriate catheter position, the pulmonary artery is occluded by balloon inflation (a pulmonary artery wedge pressure tracing is observed on the oscilloscope) and contrast media (usually 5 to 12 cc) is injected through the catheter's distal lumen. Some investigators believe Hypaque produces more vasoreactivity than Conray (54). Others have added 1.5 ml of 2% lidocaine to attenuate the cough induced by the contrast media (53). These bedside angiograms have been performed safely with no morbidity or mortality (47, 50, 52, 53). The criteria for a positive study have been the presence of an intraluminal filling defect and/or a sharp cut-off of an opacified artery (52, 53).

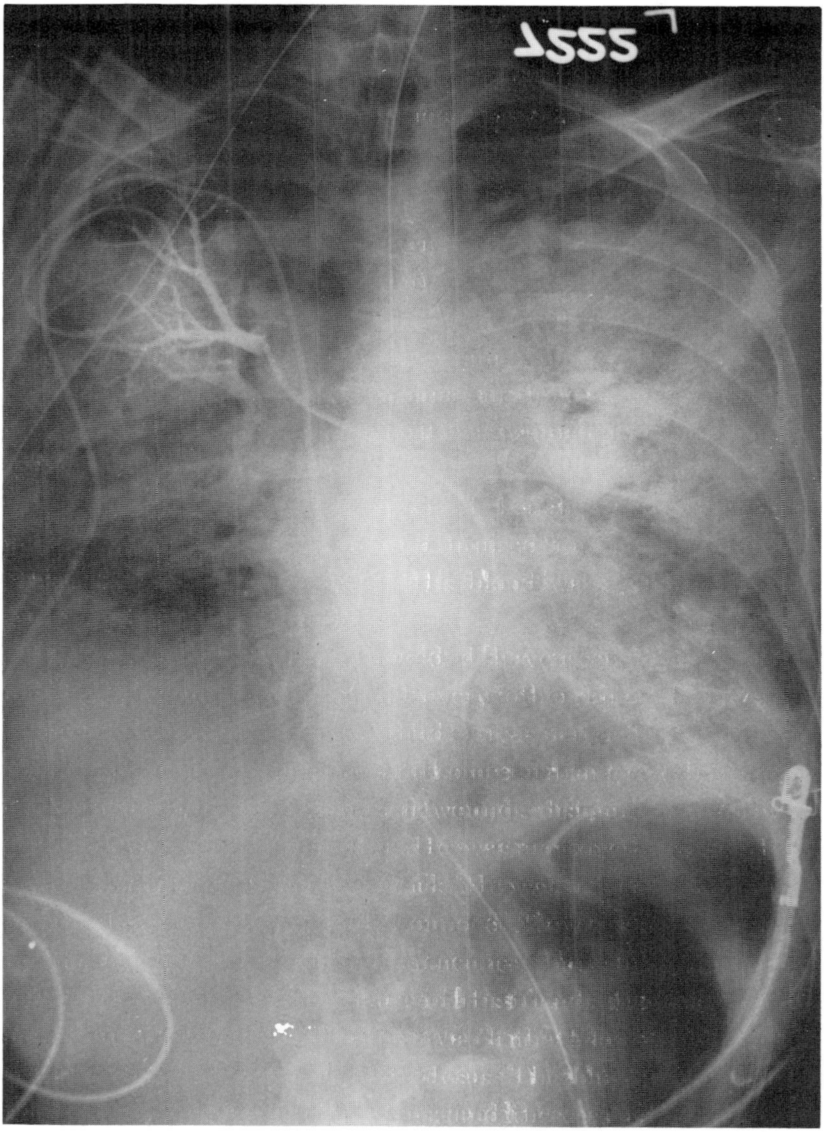

Figure 5.12. A bedside balloon occclusion pulmonary angiogram. There is no evidence of a filling defect or a cutoff of any of the arteries. The pulmonary veins are also visualized.

Pulmonary artery catheters are most frequently directed into the lower lobes of the lung presumably because of the same increased blood flow that causes pulmonary emboli to be found in the lower lobes. In addition, pulmonary emboli are commonly multiple and noted bilaterally. This pathophysiology is the basis for the usefulness of bedside balloon occlusion angiography. Of the 24 patients who have undergone bedside wedge arteriography with confirmation by autopsy, standard arteriography, or lung scan, eleven were positive, six negative, five false positive, and two false negative (50, 52, 53, 55). Therefore, this procedure can not be considered the gold standard and its limitations must be recognized. Bedside wedge angiography yields a static view of a single peripheral lobule. It is impractical to study the entire pulmonary vasculature at the bedside of a critically ill patient. If all areas of the pulmonary vasculature are not visualized, however, the study can not be considered complete and the patient may have a false negative result. In addition, caution must be exercised in interpreting the defects demonstrated by this technique (52, 53). Not all defects are caused by pulmonary emboli. An abrupt cut-off can be simulated by the different filling rates of the various pulmonary artery branches. We have attempted to avoid this problem by repeating the study and making sure that all defects are persistent. An abscess with secondary mechanical distortion of the pulmonary vessels can also cause a false positive study (53). Other limitations include the fact that if emboli are present, the flow may be greater to areas without emboli. The flotation catheter would then have a greater chance of being placed in a portion of the lung without emboli. It must also be remembered that the catheter itself may be the source of emboli. Balloon occlusion angiography may also cause balloon rupture and pulmonary hemorrhage although these complications have not yet been reported.

In conclusion, a large study to evaluate the advantages and disadvantages of bedside wedge arteriography has not been performed. The potential of this technique, therefore, remains to be elucidated. For the present, we do not advocate the routine use of balloon occlusion angiography, but in certain clinical circumstances it may add useful information and aid in the care of the critically ill.

The present patient had scleroderma and restrictive pulmonary disease for several years. The gastrointestinal hypomotility was most likely secondary to scleroderma, and the patient was therefore at a high risk for aspiration. However, the patient's underlying pulmonary disorder and constant bed rest rendered him a set up for pulmonary emboli. The etiology of the acute respiratory distress was not clear. Aspiration was believed to be the most likely cause, but the patient was receiving central hyperalimentation and had not been fed for several hours prior to the episode of dyspnea. Because of the extremely abrupt nature of the event, the hemoptysis, and the marked hypoxia, the diagnosis of pulmonary emboli was also seriously considered. The pulmonary hypertension and pulmonary artery diastolic pressure-pulmonary artery wedge pressure gradient of more than 5 mm Hg may have been due to an embolic event but may also have been present for months secondary to the patient's interstitial fibrosis. In addition, the hemoptysis may also have been due to the patient's underlying pulmonary disease. The severe hypoxia was consistent with an embolic event, but patients with chronic pulmonary disorders usually hyperventilate in the face of pulmonary emboli and typically do not hypoventilate (56). The development of the adult respiratory distress syndrome (ARDS) secondary to the presumed aspiration three days earlier was also a possibility, but ARDS usually occurs much sooner after the inciting event.

Because of the high suspicion of pulmonary emboli in this patient, the fact that the equipment for standard angiography was broken, and the fact that a pulmonary artery catheter was already in position, a balloon occlusion angiogram was performed. As can be seen in Figure 5.12, there were no intraluminal filling defects or cut-offs of any vessels. Interestingly, the catheter was wedged in the right upper lobe rather than the lower lobe. This is not a common event and may have been secondary to the patient's previously abnormal vasculature or pulmonary emboli that were present in the lower lobes. Despite the negative wedge angiogram, the physicians treated the patient with intravenous heparin. This was done because of the clinical suspicion that pulmonary emboli may have been present and because only one view rather than the entire pulmonary vasculature was observed. Over the next 24 hours the patient developed diffuse bilateral infiltrates, severe shock, and died. Autopsy findings revealed interstitial fibrosis, bilateral hemorrhagic pneumonia, and the adult respiratory distress syndrome. These findings were believed to be secondary to aspiration. No evidence of pulmonary emboli was noted.

PATIENT 11: AIR EMBOLI DURING NEUROSURGERY/ Bradley H. Ruben

A 65-year-old man was brought to the emergency room after falling from an elevation of 4 feet, striking the back of his head. On admission the patient had disconjugate gaze, was stuporous, and was arousable only to vigorous stimulation. There was no past medical history. Skull x-rays revealed a right occipital fracture with extension to the foramen magnum. Computerized axial tomography revealed a high density lesion in the vermis with extension to the right cerebellar hemisphere. There was no hydrocephalus or blood in the ventricular system. A diagnosis of a traumatic cerebellar hematoma was made. The patient was taken to the operating room for an exploration of the posterior fossa and evacuation of the hematoma.

An arterial line and central venous pressure catheter were inserted and the patient was anesthetized and placed in the sitting position. A Doppler monitoring device was positioned over the precordium. Its proper position was confirmed by the alteration in Doppler sounds when 1 ml of air was infused. After dissection and elevation of the paraspinous and occipital musculature, the fracture was noted to extend through the transverse sinus on the right side. While the occipital bone was being removed, the patient became acutely hypotensive. This hypotensive episode coincided with the development of air as noted by the Doppler device. While the surgical field was being packed, approximately 15 ml of air was withdrawn through the CVP catheter. The patient received 100%

oxygen at this time. The blood pressure slowly returned to normal and no further air could be detected by the Doppler device. During this episode there was no change in the central venous pressure. Surgery commenced once more but hypotension recurred when evidence of air in the precordium was again noted with the Doppler device. A small amount of air was again evacuated from the central line and the patient continued to receive 100% oxygen. With return of the blood pressure, the surgery was finally completed uneventfully. With the exception of the transverse sinus, no other obvious source of air entrainment was noted. Postoperatively, the patient continued to be stuporous. Repeat tomography revealed only air in the area of the craniectomy. The patient died approximately 3 weeks postoperatively secondary to pulmonary complications. He had never regained consciousness.

Discussion

Although there is always the potential for intraoperative cardiovascular collapse when elective anesthetics are given, there are few circumstances in which it is expected. Surgery performed in the seated position is such a situation and the anesthesiologist must, therefore, anticipate this complication. The most common types of procedures performed in this position are neurosurgical, that is, posterior fossa explorations and high posterior cervical laminectomies.

When the operative site is above the level of the heart, venous air embolism is a potential hazard. Cardiovascular collapse can occur if sufficient air is entrained in the right ventricle, thus causing an air-lock and consequent acute lack of right heart output (57). Venous plexuses and venous sinuses exposed during the operative dissection are the probable source of air emboli. In the clinical setting, air emboli most frequently occur as a steady stream of small air bubbles in the circulation (58). Whereas a large bolus of air can cause an air-lock in the right ventricle, the slow infusion of air causes bubbles to be dispersed throughout the cardiopulmonary circulation (57). Small air bubbles lodge in peripheral branches of the pulmonary circulation and cause mechanical obstruction as well as reflex pulmonary vasoconstriction which result in increased pulmonary artery pressures and wasted ventilation (58). When air entrainment is slow, cardiovascular collapse probably develops either from occlusion of the pulmonary outflow tract and/or from acute right heart failure. Because of this potential for air emboli to develop in patients undergoing surgery in the seated position, a central line is always placed so that aspiration of air is possible.

A number of monitoring tools have been developed for the detection of air during these neurosurgical procedures. It is believed that if air can be detected early enough, the operative site can be packed by the surgeon and open venous vessels can be occluded before more air enters the circulation. Although there are several methods for detecting venous air, many such as a precipitous rise in CVP or a "mill wheel" murmur heard through an esophageal stethoscope, occur only after large quantities of air have entered the circulation. It is extremely useful to be able to note the development of small amounts of air so that preventive measures can be instituted prior to the accumulation of large amounts of air and the ensuing hypotension.

The methods to detect air emboli and their hemodynamic consequences include the Doppler ultrasound unit, the pulmonary artery catheter, and the capnograph, which monitors end-tidal carbon dioxide (59). The Doppler is the most sensitive method to detect air emboli. It is therefore advocated as the minimum monitoring device required to reduce complications due to air emboli (60). If correctly positioned over the precordium, the Doppler can document bubbles smaller than 1 ml passing through the right atrium. Using this method, a 30% to 40% incidence of venous air embolism occurs during seated neurosurgical procedures (61). Unfortunately, the Doppler frequently detects air emboli that are clinically insignificant and may not detect all instances of clinically significant air entrainment (61). In addition, the Doppler can not quantitate the severity of circulatory impairment.

Monitoring the end-tidal CO_2 fraction is less sensitive than the Doppler device (59). It is a noninvasive technique that can alert the anesthesiologist to the entrainment of air which is sufficient to effect the pulmonary circulation before deterioration of the systemic circulation occurs. Air in the pulmonary circulation will cause ventilation-perfusion inequalities with consequent decreases in CO_2 elimination. With absorption of the pulmonary capillary air, ventilation-perfusion inequalities correct and end-tidal CO_2 returns towards the pre-existing values. Therefore, unlike the Doppler device, end-tidal CO_2 monitoring can reflect the relative severity of air emboli and can indicate when the condition is abating. Because of the high costs, however, capnographic monitoring is generally limited to busy neuro-anesthesia services.

The sensitivity of monitoring pulmonary artery pressure appears to be intermediate to Doppler and end-tidal CO_2 monitoring (62). The pulmonary artery catheter detects pulmonary hypertension in only 40% of the Doppler discovered air emboli (62). This is because the overly sensitive Doppler detects clinically insignificant events. On the other hand, changes in end-tidal CO_2 may occur only in those patients with extreme changes in pulmonary artery pressure. The presence of air in the pulmonary circulation causes pulmonary vasoconstriction, obstruction to flow, and pulmonary hypertension. Pulmonary artery pressure monitoring can promptly identify clinically significant air emboli and reflects the severity of these emboli (62). Successful treatment at the surgical site can be ascertained by the rapid return of the pulmonary artery pressure to baseline. Central venous pressure is of no diagnostic value during air emboli as minimal changes in CVP may not reflect the marked variations in pulmonary artery pressure.

Another benefit of the pulmonary artery catheter is its utility in determining the correct time to reinstitute nitrous oxide anesthesia. Because nitrous oxide is a very rapidly diffusible gas, the size of an air embolus or any residual air will rapidly increase in the presence of nitrous oxide. As previously noted, after a period of clinically significant air emboli with an increase in pulmonary artery pressures, pulmonary artery pressures decrease when air entrainment ceases and when air bubbles in the pulmonary circulation are no longer clinically significant. If nitrous oxide is reinstituted before resuming surgery and pulmonary artery pressures rise again, residual air is probably still present in the pulmonary circulation. Surgery should be delayed until pulmonary pressures no longer increase with nitrous oxide (62). Therefore, pulmonary artery pressure monitoring during certain neurosurgical procedures can be an extremely useful clinical practice.

A foramen ovale that is anatomically open but functionally closed has been termed a "probe patent foramen ovale." Its incidence in the general population is reported to be 20-30% (63). If right atrial pressure exceeds left atrial pressure, blood and air could flow from the right to the left atrium. The potential hazard of systemic air embolization is then present (64). It has been noted that after a patient has been anesthetized and moved from the supine position to the sitting position, the pulmonary artery wedge pressure (PWP)—right atrial pressure (RAP) difference decreases (65). After 1 hour of surgery, 50% of patients develop RAP greater than PWP (65). Thus, the potential for the development of systemic air embolism is present in these patients. If RAP exceeds left atrial pressure (LAP; or PWP) when placing the patient in the seated position, thought should be given to performing the surgical procedure in either the lateral decubitus or prone position.

In conclusion, the pulmonary artery catheter has been found to be a valuable diagnostic and therapeutic tool during surgery in the seated position. It is a safe, reliable, and versatile technique which can detect clinically significant episodes of air emboli, quantitate the severity of the condition, and identify successful therapeutic interventions. It also affords a route for removing air from the right heart and pulmonary artery (62) and may be used to determine the best operative position for the patient. Although no data exists comparing the complications of surgery in the seated position with and without the use of the pulmonary artery catheter, it is our belief that the benefits of its use outweigh the risks. If a pulmonary artery catheter had been placed preoperatively in the present patient and pulmonary hypertension secondary to air emboli had been noted and treated, the hypotensive episode may have been avoided.

REFERENCES

1. Stein, L., Beraud, J. J., Morissette, M., Da Luz, P., Weil, M. H., and Shubin, H. 1975. Pulmonary edema during volume infusion. Circulation 52:483-489.
2. Weiss, R. B., and Muggia, F. M. 1980. Cytoxic drug induced pulmonary disease: Update. 1980. Am. J. Med. 68:259-266.

3. Killip, T., and Kimball, J. T. 1967. Treatment of myocardial infarction in a coronary care unit. Am. J. Cardiol. 20:457-464.
4. Forrester, J. S., Diamond, G., Chatterjee, K., and Swan, H. J. C. 1976. Medical therapy of acute myocardial infarction by application of hemodynamic subsets. N. Engl. J. Med. 295:1356-1362 and 1404-1413.
5. Beta-Blocker Heart Attack Trial Research Group. 1982. A randomized trial of propranolol in patients with acute myocardial infarction. JAMA 247:1707-1714.
6. McHugh, T. J., Forrester, J. S., Adler, L., Zion, D., and Swan, H. J. C. 1972. Pulmonary vascular congestion in acute myocardial infarction: Hemodynamic and radiologic correlations. Ann. Intern. Med. 76:29-33.
7. Crexells, C., Chatterjee, K., Forrester, J. S., Dikshit, K., and Swan, H. J. C. 1973. Optimal level of filling pressure in the left side of the heart in acute myocardial infarction. N. Engl. J. Med. 289:1263-1266.
8. Dikshit, K., Vyden, J. K., Forrester, J. S., Chatterjee, K., Prakash, R., and Swan, H. J. C. 1973. Renal and extrarenal hemodynamic effects of furosemide in congestive heart failure after acute myocardial infarction. N. Engl. J. Med. 288:1087-1090.
9. Marcus, F. I. 1980. Use of digitalis in acute myocardial infarction. Circulation 62:17-19.
10. Forrester, J. S., Diamond, G. A., and Swan, H. J. C. 1977. Correlative classification of clinical and hemodynamic function after acute myocardial infarction. Am. J. Cardiol. 39:137-145.
11. Miller, R. R., Awan, N. A., Joye, J. A., Maxwell, K. S., DeMaria, A. N., Amsterdam, E. A., and Mason, D. T. 1977. Combined dopamine and nitroprusside therapy in congestive heart failure. Circulation 55:881-884.
12. Meister, S. G., and Helfant, R. H. 1972. Rapid bedside differentiation of ruptured interventricular septum from acute mitral insufficiency. N. Engl. J. Med. 287:1024-1025.
13. Fuchs, R. M., Heuser, R. R., Yin, F. C. P., and Brinker, J. A. 1982. Limitations of pulmonary wedge v-waves in diagnosing mitral regurgitation. Am. J. Cardiol. 49:849-854.
14. Cohn, J. N., and Franciosa, J. A. 1977. Vasodilator therapy of cardiac failure. N. Engl. J. Med. 297:27-31.
15. Packman, M. I., and Rackow, E. C. 1981. Optimum left heart filling pressure during fluid challenge of patients with septic shock. Crit. Care Med. 9(Abstract): 234.
16. Skillman, J. J. 1976. The role of albumin and oncotically active fluids in shock. Crit. Care Med. 4:55-61.
17. Shoemaker, W. C. 1976. Comparison of the relative effectiveness of whole blood transfusions and various types of fluid therapy in resuscitation. Crit. Care Med. 4:71-78.
18. Virgilio, R. W., Smith, D. E., and Zarins, C. K. 1979. Balanced electrolyte solutions: Experimental and clinical studies. Crit. Care Med. 7:98-106.
19. Lowe, R. J., Moss, G. S., Jilek, J., and Levine, H. D. 1979. Crystalloid versus colloid in the etiology of pulmonary failure after trauma—a randomized trial in man. Crit. Care Med. 7:107-112.
20. Weil, M. H., Henning, R. J., and Puri, V. K. 1979. Colloid oncotic pressure: Clinical significance. Crit. Care Med. 7:113-116.
21. Shoemaker, W. C., and Hauser, C. J. 1979. Critique of crystalloid versus colloid therapy in shock and shock lung. Crit. Care Med. 7:117-124.

22. Rackow, E. C., Fein, I. A., and Leppo, J. 1977. Colloid osmotic pressure as a prognostic indicator of pulmonary edema and mortality in the critically ill. Chest 72:709-713.
23. Weil, M. H., and Nishijima, H. 1978. Cardiac output in bacterial shock. Am. J. Med. 64:920-922.
24. Sibbald, W. J., Paterson, A. M., Holliday, R. L., Anderson, R. A., Lobb, T. R., and Duff, J. H. 1978. Pulmonary hypertension in sepsis. Chest 73:583-591.
25. Kreger, B. E., Craven, D. E., and McCabe, W. R. 1980. Gram-negative bacteremia, Am. J. Med. 68:344-355.
26. Jardin, F., Eveleigh, M. C., Gurdjian, F., Delille, F., and Margairaz, A. 1979. Venous admixture in human septic shock. Circulation 60:155-159.
27. Brigham, K. L., Woolverton, W., Blake, L., and Staub, N. C. 1974. Increased sheep lung vascular permeability caused by *Pseudomonas* bacteremia. J. Clin. Invest. 54:792-804.
28. Sprung, C. L., Rackow, E. C., Fein, I. A., Jacob, A. I., and Isikoff, S. K. 1981. The spectrum of pulmonary edema: Differentiation of cardiogenic, intermediate, and noncardiogenic forms of pulmonary edema. Am. Rev. Respir. Dis. 124:718-722.
29. Unger, K. M., Shibel, E. M., and Moser, K. M. 1975. Detection of left ventricular failure in patients with adult respiratory distress syndrome. Chest 67: 8-13.
30. Cassidy, S. S., and Mitchell, J. H. 1981. Effects of positive pressure breathing on right and left ventricular preload and afterload. Fed. Proc. 40:2178-2181.
31. Suter, P. M., Fairley, H. B., and Isenberg, M. D. 1975. Optimum end-expiratory airway pressure in patients with acute pulmonary failure. N. Engl. J. Med. 292:284-289.
32. Gallagher, T. J., Civetta, J. M., and Kirby, R. R. 1978. Terminology update: Optimal PEEP. Crit. Care Med. 6:323-326.
33. Sibbald, W. J., Driedger, A. A., Moffat, J. D., Myers, M. L., Reid, B. A., and Holliday, R. L. 1981. Pulmonary microvascular clearance of radiotracers in human cardiac and noncardiac pulmonary edema. J. Appl. Physiol. 50:1337-1347.
34. Hammerschmidt, D. E., Weaver, L. J., Hudson, L. D., Craddock, P. R., and Jacob, H. S. 1980. Association of complement activation and elevated plasma—C5a with adult respiratory distress syndrome. Lancet 1:947-949.
35. Sibbald, W. J., Anderson, R. R., Reid, B., Holliday, R. L., and Driedger, A. A., 1981. Alveolo-capillary permeability in human septic ARDS. Effect of high-dose corticosteroid therapy. Chest 79:133-142.
36. Calvin, J. E., Driedger, A. A., and Sibbald, W. J. 1981. Does the pulmonary capillary wedge pressure predict left ventricular preload in critically ill patients? Crit. Care Med. 9:437-443.
37. Robotham, J. L., Lixfeld, W., Holland, L., MacGregor, D., Bromberger-Barnea, B., Permutt, S., and Rabson, J. L. 1980. The effects of positive end-expiratory pressure on right and left ventricular performance. Am. Rev. Respir. Dis. 121:677-683.
38. Danek, S. J., Lynch, J. P., Weg, J. G., and Dantzker, D. R. 1980. The dependence of oxygen uptake on oxygen delivery in the adult respiratory distress syndrome. Am. Rev. Respir. Dis. 122:387-395.
39. Prys-Roberts, C. 1979. Hypertension and anesthesia—fifty years on. Anesthesiology 50:281-284.
40. Tarhan, S., Moffit, E. A., Sessler, A. D., Douglas, W. W., and Taylor, W. F. 1973. Risk of anesthesia and surgery in patients with chronic bronchitis and chronic obstructive pulmonary disease. Surgery 74:720-726.

41. Foex, P. 1980. Preoperative assessment of patients with cardiac disease. Int. Anesthes. Clin. 18:81-109.
42. Powers, J. H. (ed). 1968. Surgery of the Aged and Debilitated Patient. p. 205. W. B. Saunders Company, Philadelphia and London.
43. Del Guercio, L. M., and Cohn, S. D. 1980. Monitoring operative risk in the elderly. JAMA 243:1350-1355.
44. Robinson, B. F. 1967. Relation of heart rate and systolic blood pressure to the onset of pain in angina pectoris. Circulation 35:1073-1083.
45. Mangano, D. T. 1980. Monitoring pulmonary artery pressure in coronary artery disease. Anesthesiology 53:364-370.
46. Kaplan, J. A., and Wells, P. H. 1981. Early diagnosis of myocardial ischemia using the pulmonary arterial catheter. Anesth. Analg. 60:789-793.
47. Wilson, J. E., and Bynum, L. J. 1976. An improved pulmonary angiographic technque using a balloon-tipped catheter. Am. Rev. Respir. Dis. 114:1137-1144.
48. Bell, A. L., Shimomura, S., Guthrie, W. J., Hempel, H. F., Fitzpatrick, H. F., and Begg, C. F. 1959. Wedge pulmonary arteriography. Radiology 73: 566-574.
49. Stein, P. D. 1971. Wedge arteriography for the identification of pulmonary emboli in small vessels. Am. Heart J. 82:618-623.
50. Loop, J. W., Archer, G., and Northrop, C. H. 1975. Bedside pulmonary arteriography. Radiology 114:469-471.
51. Alsbrook, E. H., Comer, P. B., Gibson, R. L., and Reidy, J. F. 1976. Pulmonary angiography via an indwelling four-channel Swan-Ganz catheter. Crit. Care Med. 4:320-322.
52. Orta, D. A., Eisen, S., Yergin, B. M., and Olsen, G. N. 1979. Segmental pulmonary angiography in the critically ill patient using a flow-directed catheter. Chest 76:269-273.
53. Dougherty, J. E., LaSala, A. F., and Fieldman, A. 1980. Bedside pulmonary angiography utilizing an existing Swan-Ganz catheter. Chest 77:43-46.
54. Lefcoe, M. S. 1981. Opacification of pulmonary veins during wedge angiography. Crit. Care Med. 9:128-129.
55. Greene, R., Zapol, W. M., Snider, M. T., Reid, L., Snow, R., O'Connell, R. S., and Novelline, R. A. 1981. Early bedside detection of pulmonary vascular occlusion during acute respiratory failure. Am. Rev. Respir. Dis. 124:593-601.
56. Lippmann, M., and Fein, A. 1981. Pulmonary embolism in the patient with chronic obstructive pulmonary disease. Chest 79:39-42.
57. Adornato, D. C., Gildenberg, P. L., Ferrario, C. M., Smart, J., and Frost, E. A. M. 1978. Pathophysiology of intravenous air embolism in dogs. Anesthesiology 49:120-127.
58. Munson, E. S., Paul, W. C., Perry, J. C., de Padua, C. B., and Rhoton, A. L. 1975. Early detection of venous air embolism using a Swan-Ganz catheter. Anesthesiology 42:223-226.
59. English, J. B., Westenskow, D., Hodges, M. R., and Stanley, T. H. 1978. Comparison of venous air embolism-monitoring methods in supine dogs. Anesthesiology 48:425-429.
60. Edmonds-Seal, J., and Maroon, J. C. 1969. Air-embolism diagnosed with ultrasound. Anesthesia 24:438-440.
61. Michenfelder, J. D., Miller, R. H., and Gronert, G. A. 1972. Evaluation of an ultrasonic device (Doppler) for the diagnosis of air embolism. Anesthesiology 36:164-167.
62. Marshall, W. K., and Bedford, R. F. 1980. Use of pulmonary artery catheter for

detection and treatment of venous air embolism: A prospective study in man. Anesthesiology 52:131-134.

63. Edwards, J. E. 1960. Interatrial communication. Pathology of the heart. Gould, S. E. (ed). pp 260-261. Charles C Thomas, Springfield, IL.
64. Gronert, G. A., Messick, J. M., Cuchiara, R. F., and Michenfelder, J. D. 1979. Paradoxical air embolism from a patent foramen ovale. Anesthesiology 50:548-549.
65. Perkins-Pearson, N. A. K., Marshall, W. K., and Bedford, R. F. 1981. Atrial pressures and air embolism in the seated position. Anesthesiology 55:A236 (Supplement).

Appendix: Abbreviations

AFB acid fast bacillus
AMI acute myocardial infarction
AML acute myelogenous leukemia
$avDO_2$ arteriovenous oxygen content difference
ARDS adult respiratory distress syndrome
BP blood pressure
BSA body surface area
BUN blood urea nitrogen
CaO_2 arterial oxygen content
CcO_2 capillary oxygen content
CDC Centers for Disease Control
CI cardiac index
CO cardiac output
COD coefficient of oxygen delivery
COP colloid osmotic pressure
CPAP continuous positive airway pressure
CPE cardiogenic pulmonary edema
CPK creatine phosphokinase
CVA costovertebral angle
cvO_2 central venous oxygen saturation
CvO_2 mixed venous oxygen content
CVP central venous pressure
DBP diastolic blood pressure
DPG diphosphoglyceric acid
ECG electrocardiogram
FIO_2 inspired oxygen concentration
Hct hematocrit
Hgb hemoglobin
HR heart rate
ICU intensive care unit
IVC inferior vena cava

K_f filtration coefficient
LAP left atrial pressure
LDH lactic dehydrogenase
LVDP left ventricular diastolic pressure
LVEDP left ventricular end-diastolic pressure
LVEDV left ventricular end-diastolic volume
LVSW left ventricular stroke work
MAP mean arterial pressure
MPAP mean pulmonary artery pressure
NCPE noncardiogenic pulmonary edema
NYHA New York Heart Association
O_2 oxygen
PA pulmonary artery
PADP pulmonary artery diastolic pressure
PAEDP pulmonary artery end-diastolic pressure
PAO,PAOP pulmonary artery occlusion pressure
PASP pulmonary artery systolic pressure
Pc capillary hydrostatic pressure
pCO_2 arterial carbon dioxide tension
PCP pulmonary capillary pressure
PCW pulmonary capillary wedge pressure
PEEP positive end-expiratory pressure
Pis hydrostatic pressure in the interstitial space
π_c capillary osmotic pressure
π_{is} osmotic pressure in the interstitial space
PMI point of maximal impulse
pO_2 arterial oxygen tension
PVC premature ventricular contraction(s)
$pvCO_2$ mixed venous carbon dioxide tension
pvO_2 mixed venous oxygen tension
PVR pulmonary vascular resistance
PWP pulmonary artery wedge pressure
Qs/Qt veno-arterial admixture or pulmonary shunt
RAP right atrial pressure
RVSW right ventricular stroke work
SBP systolic blood pressure
SGOT serum glutamic oxalacetic transaminase

SGPT serum glutamic pyruvic transaminase

SI stroke index

σ reflection coefficient

SV stroke volume

SVI stroke volume index

SVC superior vena cava

svO_2 mixed venous oxygen saturation

SVR systemic vascular resistance

VO_2 oxygen consumption

VSD ventricular septal defect

WBC white blood cell count

Index